THE TLC STORY
Mild Dementia

A Guide for Caregivers of Loved Ones in the Mild Stage of Alzheimer's and Related Dementia Diseases

By
Tom Connolly

Copyright 2020 Thomas Connolly

Title: The TLC Story – Mild Dementia:

Subtitle: A Guide for Caregivers of Loved Ones in the Mild Stage of Alzheimer's and Related Dementia Diseases

Author: Connolly, Tom

Author website: www.tlc4dementia.com

Published in 2020 by: Dementia Caregiving Using TLC.

First edition dated 2020. Printed on Demand and bound in the United States.

Library of Congress Control Number: 2020900138

International Standard Book Numbers:

Paperback book ISBN: 978-1-7344064-0-5

Digital/electronic book ISBN: 978-1-7344064-1-2

Author-generated Library of Congress Catalog Information and Numbers:

Senile dementia – Patients – Home care. RC521 .C67 2020

Dewey Decimal Number 616.83 .C67 – dc23 (Dementia – Patients –Care)

Dedication: This book is dedicated to you, the previous, current or future caregiver. It is intended to help you become proficient in providing Tender Loving Care to a loved one living with dementia.

ACKNOWLEDGMENTS

I would like to thank our children, my family members and friends, Laura's family and her close personal friends, our neighbors, social and duplicate bridge players, church members, retired military members and their wives, retired telephone pioneers and their wives, friends, writing group members, my author friends and our personal physician. From these people and many written sources, I eventually became proficient in providing Laura with Tender Loving Care. It is the absolute minimum a loved one living with dementia deserves. My purpose is to help others work toward this goal.

Victoria Rosendahl edited this book. In fact, she suggested we divide the original long book into separate mild, moderate and severe stages. This provides specific and focused application to caregivers with loved ones in each of those stages. Her comments were insightful and inspiring and I'm confident she helped make it a better book than it was originally. If you are looking for an editor, Victoria can be reached at victoria@therosendahlmethod.com.

The book cover design and interior text formatting of both the paperback and eBook versions were completed by the EbookPbook Company. The performance of the Jason and Vidya team was exceptional. They have my highest recommendation and may be reached at jason@ebookpbook.com.

Limitation of Liability and Disclaimer of Warranty Information:

The information and advice contained in this work is relating to improving the home health care of loved ones living with dementia. It is not intended as medical advice or as a substitute for medical advice or counseling by physicians, experts or professionals in this area. The information should be evaluated and considered as a possible supplement to the guidance and care of a physician or another trained health professional. At this time, it is generally acknowledged that there is no cure for dementia diseases, nor is there a treatment that will slow the progression of these eventually fatal diseases. No one has all the answers, especially the author of this work. The advice and recommendations contained in this work may not be suitable for a specific individual's situation. The information is not intended to substitute for expert medical advice and treatment. It is offered to help caregivers make informed choices because each individual's needs for care are unique and different. The author encourages caregivers to regularly seek medical expertise from physicians and other qualified health care practitioners in all matters that require medical attention so that an optimum individual treatment plan can be developed.

While the author has used his best efforts in preparing this work, the author makes no representations or warranties with respect to the accuracy or completeness of the information presented. The author encourages all readers to consult with medical professionals as appropriate.

In the event that any information in this work is contrary to information, advice or guidance provided by a physician or other qualified health care practitioner, then that professional's advice and guidance should be followed as it is based on the unique characteristics of the individual under the supervised care of that professional.

TABLE OF CONTENTS

Acknowledgments   v
Introduction   xi

Chapter 1   The Big Picture   1
Chapter 2   Dispelling Common Myths About Dementia   8
Chapter 3   What is NOT Dementia   16
Chapter 4   What Exactly is Dementia?   25
Chapter 5   What Exactly is Alzheimer's Disease?   30
Chapter 6   What are Some Other Dementia Diseases?   40
Chapter 7   Cognitive (Communicational Types) Early
             Warning Signs   47
Chapter 8   Cognitive (but less complex)
             Early Warning Signs   54
Chapter 9   Cognitive (but more complex)
             Early Warning Signs   63
Chapter 10   Physical Early Warning Signs   73
Chapter 11   Emotional Early Warning Signs   83
Chapter 12   Do It Yourself Mild Dementia Diagnosis   89
Chapter 13   The Right to Avoid a Dementia Diagnosis   99
Chapter 14   The Right to Obtain an Accurate Dementia
             Diagnosis   111
Chapter 15   Telling the Diagnosis   127
Chapter 16   The Right to Personal Privacy   136
Chapter 17   The Right to Exercise Denial   144
Chapter 18   Advance Planning   150
Chapter 19   Words Matter   167
Chapter 20   TLC Action Plan Going Forward   178
Chapter 21   Epilogue (Preview of Moderate Dementia)   196

INTRODUCTION

"God gave us burdens ... he also gave us shoulders."
– Yiddish Proverb

"TLC" is a common language abbreviation for Tender Loving Care. It is also the monogram used by Laura to personalize our guest bedroom pillows. It is our initials, Thomas and Laura Connolly. The TLC Story is both the title and the theme for this book.

It is a story of our love and how the love we had for each other was strengthened and enhanced by the dreaded diseases called dementia. Using the plural "diseases" was not a mistake. Laura had Alzheimer's disease dementia, Vascular disease dementia, and Lewy Body disease dementia. Her diagnosis was mixed dementia.

She hit the jackpot for the wide spectrum of challenging behaviors that dementia causes. Was it more difficult for her than me? Was it more difficult for me than her? I benefited from learning about dementia and will now share that knowledge with you.

You will benefit from reading The TLC Story.

Laura is deceased now but still lives on in both my conscious and subconscious mind. Consequently, in this book I often use the present tense to give you my thoughts. My fingers use the keyboard of a laptop to produce the written pages, but it is Laura's voice that tells me what to write. Her nonstop verbal patter in my brain motivates me to write, revise, and rewrite every day. If this book is superb, it is because of her. She lived the motto, "If it's worth doing, it's worth doing well."

When did the TLC story start? The stages are called Mild, Moderate and Severe. How long was each stage? When did the TLC story end?

I do not know exactly when Laura's mild cognitive impairment started, but I have some reasonable suspicions. Medical authorities agree that Alzheimer's disease starts long before any symptoms become apparent, possibly as much as a decade or two. This is called preclinical Alzheimer's disease. Since writing this book about Laura's mild stage, I have given much thought about when her symptoms actually were apparent to me.

When Laura worked in mid-life, she was primarily in retail sales because she could arrange her schedule to work when the children were in school or when I was home from work to care for them. Laura was extremely successful at every job she had, including retail sales. When working, she always performed at her best. Laura was always the troubleshooter or "go to" person when management or a co-worker had a problem. In her final employment at a nationwide, AT&T retail sales store, she really excelled. Almost every month, she was highest in sales for the District; in many quarters, she was highest in sales for the State; and a few times she was highest in sales for the Nation. She brought home many sales awards from her company. Laura loved to talk, meet new people and help customers find the correct product. Customers loved to buy from her, often waiting to be helped by Laura when they returned for additional items. She had many sales due to referrals from satisfied customers. However, if a coworker's job was in jeopardy due to poor sales, Laura would ring up her personal sales using the coworker's identification number until the supervisor relaxed the pressure. The entire sales team loved Laura, tried to follow her example, and learned from her sales techniques. She refused any consideration for a promotion to management because she enjoyed the direct customer contact.

When Laura was 53 or 54, she started to complain to me about her co-workers. This was unusual for her because she was always in her comfort zone with both customers and co-workers. This issue really got my attention when Laura mentioned quitting her job because of animosity between herself and some of her colleagues. Since she was close to seven years of service ... which was the then-current requirement to be entitled to a vested pension ... I strongly discouraged any thought of her quitting. About the same time, as our daughter was preparing to leave home to attend a university, Laura became somewhat depressed. This was also unusual for her. She was a life-long happy, up-beat person.

We would be empty nesters – which I anticipated with pleasure – because we would gain more independence and have less parenting responsibility. About this time, Laura started to nag me about seeking a transfer to the city where our daughter would attend the university. This was also unlike her because Laura had many friends where we lived for over a decade and raised our two children. However, as luck would have it, Laura passed her seven-year service mark and, at the same time, I was fortunate to be offered a transfer to that university city. Laura was 54.

I now believe Laura's unusual behavior could have been prompted by her entering mild cognitive impairment which is a potential entry gate to dementia. Laura thrived in the university city for a time but after several years our daughter graduated from college, moved away and married. Then, Laura seemed to become bored but about that time her former company was seeking some temporary sales representatives. This would have been ideal for Laura because after the temporary job ended, she could draw unemployment compensation for the same length of time. The position would have been similar to her previous job where she excelled so I thought it was perfect.

But Laura failed the employment test! This astounded me because that test is not overly complex. Laura had passed the same test with flying colors twice in the past ten years, once for a temporary position and once for a permanent position. So, with hindsight, I now believe Laura entered mild dementia at that time, which caused her to perform poorly on the logic, reasoning, problem-solving and basic mathematics problems in that basic skills employment test. Laura was about 59 at that time.

This occurred 20 years before she died of dementia at age 79. Twelve years later when Laura was 71, she exhibited behavior which was definitely consistent with moderate dementia. At 76, Laura no longer recognized me and tried to kill the "old man" (me) who was providing care for her. Naturally, I judge this behavior to be consistent with late moderate to early severe stage dementia. To recap, I believe Laura had mild cognitive impairment for five years, mild dementia for 12 years, moderate dementia for five years and severe dementia for three years. Naturally, overlap existed among these stages. This was about half of our married life of 51 years. Thank goodness for Tender Loving Care. It helped both of us immensely.

Laura and I are neither medical practitioners nor dementia researchers. In this first book, I will detail what happened to us during the mild stage. Two more books will follow with experiences from the moderate and severe stages.

This book will not advise you on medications, specific alternative treatment plans, or specialized geriatric or dementia practitioners to consult. Laura and I have had experiences. Some good, some bad, some beautiful and some ugly. We are sharing the naked truth about living with dementia to help you know how to better deal with it using tender loving caregiving.

The focus of this book is to help you and your loved one living with dementia. It will significantly improve your understanding and knowledge level of dementia as well as providing valuable and practical caregiving tips and recommendations. By gaining coping skills, you will be able to minimize the negative aspects of caregiving, while maximizing the positive so both of you will reap benefits.

This is our story.

CHAPTER 1

The Big Picture

"There are no easy answers, but there are simple answers. We must have the courage to do what we know is morally right."
– Ronald Reagan

What does dementia look like from a bird's eye view, from fifty thousand feet up? It is always valuable to understand an overview of any problem before diving deep to understand it.

Dementia has existed for thousands of years, but is known by other names. Just a few decades ago, the symptoms of dementia were called "senility" or "hardening of the arteries."

Ancient History of Dementia

Ancient physicians in all cultures knew that an extremely aged person sometimes had afflictions that eventually rendered that person to become helpless. Pythagoras, in the 7th century B.C., divided the life cycle into numerous stages. The last two were identified as the decay of the human body and the regression of the human mental abilities. [1]

Hippocrates lived between the third and fourth centuries B.C. and called the deterioration of mind due to old age as "paranoia" and thought it was a common and normal occurrence to all those growing old. Both Plato and his student Aristotle thought of mental and cognitive decline as an unavoidable consequence of age. Cicero, in the second century B.C., suggested that an active mental life could prevent or postpone cognitive decline. [1]

In the second century A.D., Roman emperor Marcus Aurelius employed Galen of Pergamon, a Greek-born physician. Galen was a highly productive author who composed hundreds of dissertations involving medicine. He used the term "morosis" to describe dementia diseases. This word meant "mental slowness, dementia." It included loss of memory, reason and understanding. The now derogatory term "moron" comes from this word. Galen is credited with stating that people with this condition were "some in whom the knowledge of letters and other arts are totally obliterated, indeed, they can't even remember their own names." [1, 2, 3]

Now, fast forward to the present time to continue our overview. We can't have a thorough discussion of what Laura and I went through without looking at some statistics first.

Statistics

The world's population is 7.3 billion and about 50 million have dementia. About every three seconds, someone in the world is diagnosed with dementia, a total of about 10 million people each year. [4, 5]

There are more people living with dementia in the world than the total population of Canada. Speaking of our northern neighbor, over 747,000 Canadians are living with dementia. [5]

The disease is a global health crisis being addressed by millions of researchers and their supporting administrative organizations/associations. Alzheimer's Disease International (ADI) has over 120 countries banded together to find a cure. [6] Alzheimer's Europe has over 40 member and provisional member countries in its organization working towards the mitigation of dementia. [7] Spanish speaking countries consolidate their efforts in the Alzheimer Ibero America organization. [8]

In the U.S., the National Institutes for Health (NIH) in Bethesda, Maryland provides leadership in all areas of health for the government's major health initiatives. The NIH budget for 2018 was $37 billion with Alzheimer's disease research weighing in at $1.8 billion. [9]

Worldwide, much research is being conducted on how to prevent, delay the onset of, and slow the progression of dementia, however, the U.S. is currently the world leader in combatting dementia. [9]

The United States population is 327 million [4] and about 5.8 million people live with dementia. This number is projected to rise to nearly 14 million by 2050. About every 65 seconds, someone in the U.S. is diagnosed with dementia, a total of about 500,000 each year. [10]

Of the millions of seniors in the U.S. living with dementia, about two-thirds are women. It is generally thought that this is because women simply live longer than men on average and because older age is the greatest risk factor for Alzheimer's. The majority of loved ones living with dementia are cared for at home, either their own home or a relative's home, by family members and friends. Proper care of loved ones living with dementia requires knowledgeable and effective caregivers. As the disease progresses, more caregiver assistance is required. About half of all caregivers are married to or living with a partner or in a long-term relationship with the loved one. About half of all caregivers are caring for a parent. [10]

The following excerpts are direct quotations from the U.S. Alzheimer's 2019 annual report:

On Caregivers

- More than 16 million Americans provide unpaid care for people with Alzheimer's or other dementias. These caregivers provided an 18.5 billion hours of care valued at nearly $234 billion.
- Eighty-three percent of the help provided to older adults in the United States comes from family caregivers, friends or other unpaid caregivers. Nearly half of all caregivers who provide help to older adults do so for someone living with Alzheimer's or another dementia.
- About one in three caregivers is age 65 or older.
- Approximately two-thirds of caregivers are women; more specifically, over one-third of caregivers are daughters.

- Alzheimer's takes a devastating toll on caregivers. Compared with caregivers of people without dementia, twice as many caregivers of those with dementia indicate substantial emotional, financial and physical difficulties. [10]

On Life Expectancies

- One in three seniors dies with multiple issues including Alzheimer's or another dementia. It kills more than breast cancer and prostate cancer combined.
- Alzheimer's disease is the sixth leading cause of death among those age 65 and older and is also a leading cause of disability and poor health.
- Between 2000 and 2017, deaths from heart disease decreased 9% while deaths from Alzheimer's increased 145%.
- Among people age 70, over 60 percent of those with Alzheimer's dementia are expected to die before the age of 80 compared with 30 percent of people without Alzheimer's, which is a rate twice as high. [10]

On Costs

- In 2019, Alzheimer's and other dementias will cost the nation $290 billion. By 2050, these costs could rise as high as $1.1 trillion.
- People living with Alzheimer's and other dementias have twice as many hospitals stays per year than other older people.
- Medicare beneficiaries with Alzheimer's or other dementias are more likely than those without dementia to have other chronic conditions such as heart disease, diabetes and kidney disease.
- Older people living with Alzheimer's or other dementias have more skilled nursing facility stays and home health care visits per year than other older people.

- People living with Alzheimer's or other dementias make up a large proportion of all elderly people who receive adult day services and nursing home care. [10]

On Aging

- Of course, both physical and mental abilities generally deteriorate over time. Some witty people call this gradual deterioration "old-timers" syndrome.
- Studies indicate that people age 65 and older survive an average of 4 to 8 years after a diagnosis of Alzheimer's dementia, yet some live as long as 20 years. This reflects the slow, insidious and uncertain progression of Alzheimer's. Of the total years they live with Alzheimer's dementia, individuals will spend an average of 40 percent of this time in dementia's most severe stage. Much of this time will be spent in a nursing home. At age 80, approximately 75 percent of people living with severe dementia are expected to live in a nursing home compared with only 4 percent of the general population at the same age. In all, an estimated two-thirds of those who die of dementia do so in nursing homes, while one-third die either at home, hospice facilities, or hospitals. [10]

Interestingly, comparing many sources and studies, I have not found any published information that provides universal agreement and an exact correlation of physical deterioration and cognitive loss due to advancing age.

The Alzheimer's Association 2019 Alzheimer's Facts and Figures; Risk Factors for Alzheimer's Dementia states this:

The percentage of loved ones living with dementia definitely increases with aging: 3 percent of people age 65-74, 17 percent of people age 75-84 and 32 percent of people age 85 or older have Alzheimer's dementia. [10]

Lisa Genova, a best-selling author and lecturer, starts her YouTube TED Talk video with an attention getter when addressing a large audience as follows: "I think we all have his hopeful expectation of living into old age. Let's project out into the future, to your future you and let's imagine that we're all 85. Now everyone look at two people. One of you probably has Alzheimer's disease. And maybe you are thinking, well OK, it won't be me. Then OK, you are probably a caregiver." [11]

Factoring in other estimates of Mild Cognitive Impairment, other diseases which also cause dementia additional to Alzheimer's and the reality that dementia is probably underdiagnosed, my personal rough guesstimate is that about 10 percent of seniors aged 65 and older, about 20 percent of seniors aged 75 and older, and about 40 percent of seniors aged 85 and older are living with dementia.

To summarize, I personally believe the prevalence of dementia about doubles every ten years until people reach age 85 or older.

Tips and Recommendations

Accept the reality that most people will have progressive neurodegenerative disease in their lifetime or will become a caregiver for a loved one living with this disease. You are not alone. Caregiving and/or being cared for is an important part of life.

Positive Affirmations

"We think sometimes that poverty is only being hungry, naked and homeless. The poverty of being unwanted, unloved and uncared for is the greatest poverty." – *Mother Theresa*

"If you want happiness for an hour – take a nap. If you want happiness for a day – go fishing. If you want happiness for a year – inherit a fortune. If you want happiness for a life time – help someone else." – *Chinese proverb*

End Notes

[1]   https://www.gerassolutions – A brief history of dementia, January 18, 2018

[2]   https://www.medcrave

[3]   MedCrave Journal of Neurosciences, Volume 4 Issue 1 – 2016

[4]   https://www.worldmeters.org

[5]   https://www.alzheimer.ca

[6]   https://alz.co.uk.research

[7]   https://www.alzheimer-europe.org

[8]   https://www.alzheimeriberoamerica.org

[9]   https://www.nia.nih.gov-alzheimers

[10] Alzheimer's Association 2019 Alzheimer's Facts and Figures; Risk Factors for Alzheimer's Dementia and https://www.org/alzheimers-dementia/facts-figures

[11] Lisa Genova, YouTube TED Talk video, "What you can do to prevent Alzheimer's." 1,454,921 views as of July 22, 2019.

CHAPTER 2

Dispelling Common Myths About Dementia

"You gain strength, courage, and confidence by every experience in which you really stop to look fear in the face. You are able to say to yourself, "I lived through this horror. I can take the next thing that comes along."
– Eleanor Roosevelt

There are numerous myths about dementia diseases and Laura and I were exposed to many of them. Because these myths are an important part of the big picture, I wanted to make sure we touch on them.

This isn't an exhaustive list. You could Google "dementia myths" and come up millions of hits. You read that right. Millions!

MYTH #1
Life for the loved one living with dementia is over. Death is close.

Wrong. Over five million people in the U.S. alone are now living with dementia and most are enjoying their lives. A caregiving focus on improving the quality of life for someone living with dementia can and will make a positive difference.

MYTH # 2
Life for the caregiver is over and life will be constantly difficult and miserable.

Wrong again. There is a host of positive actions that can be considered to ensure the caregiver has a healthy and happy life. The most important are preparedness, predictability and bondedness. Learn as much as possible about the disease to make sure you're prepared and are able to generally predict what symptoms come next. When the caregiver is bonded with the loved one, you can handle most of the issues in a reasonable and effective manner.

MYTH # 3
Since there is no cure for dementia, there is nothing that can be done. It is hopeless.

Boy, this is one of the worst myths. There are important health care general strategies, specific person-centered actions and numerous positive aspects of caregiving that can improve the quality of life for the loved one living with dementia. Laura and I found that what is good for the heart, is also good for the brain. We found that a plant-based diet, physical exercise, socialization and cognitive challenges were all important to us. And we found that medications to lower cholesterol, lower blood pressure, improve mood and manage blood sugar were also extremely important for a person living with dementia.

MYTH # 4
Dementia is a death sentence for aged people at the end of their lives.

Nope. As we stated above, over 5 million people in the U.S. and 50 million worldwide are living with dementia and not all of them are older. The focus for you as a caregiver should be on what the loved one can do.

MYTH # 5
Other diseases can be ignored if someone is diagnosed with dementia.

Here's why this myth is dangerous: Two-thirds of those living with dementia are women and have double the risk of dying from breast cancer than dementia. [1] Add in the risk of heart attacks, strokes, infectious diseases, motor vehicle accidents, drug overdoses, hospital-acquired infections and a smorgasbord of other killers, it is clear that many other factors can end a person's life before dementia enters the end stage. For the one-third of dementia sufferers who are men, their gender marks them for an earlier death than women. However, the same life-risks apply and, in many cases, even more so.

MYTH # 6
There will never be a drug that helps the symptoms of dementia.

Thankfully, that statement is just plain wrong. As of this writing, there are four U.S. approved prescription drugs that moderate the symptoms of dementia and they are used world-wide. There are also numerous prescription drugs that are used "off label" because medical practitioners have found that some drugs in particular doses do help some people with dementia. Make sure to do your homework and talk with your primary medical practitioner before using any prescription or non-prescription drug.

Most medical practitioners address the possible benefit of certain drugs or drug combinations that may lesson or moderate symptoms based on personal trial and error. Some symptoms unique to certain types of dementia diseases may be significantly reduced by certain drugs. When they are found to be beneficial, the reward may far exceed the risk.

MYTH # 7
There will never be a drug that slows or cures any type of dementia disease.

Never say never. There is a massive world-wide effort involving millions of medical professionals who study and research numerous initiatives. Eventually one or more of these initiatives, or a combination of these initiatives, will have a break-through and produce a drug, a medical procedure, or a treatment to moderate or cure specific dementia diseases. Keep believing.

MYTH # 8
Jokes about dementia are funny.

Jokes like these are just plain cruel. There is nothing funny about the physical, mental or emotional behavior of a person living with dementia. But, if you encounter a mean-spirited and heartless person who makes jokes about people having dementia or any other special needs person with birth deformities, handicaps, serious or incurable illnesses, then immediately assert yourself and set that person straight.

MYTH # 9
Reality Orientation therapy and methods is the best approach for caregivers.

If you're unfamiliar with Reality Orientation, here's how the National Institutes for Health (NIH) describes it: Reality Orientation for dementia...operates through the presentation of orientation information (e.g. time, place and person-related) which is thought to provide the person with a greater understanding of their surroundings, possibly resulting in an improved sense of control and self-esteem. [1]

We found that Reality Orientation therapy and methods may be used with extreme caution and sensitivity in the mild stage and possibly early in the moderate stage. After progressing to later in the moderate stage and throughout the severe stage, Reality Orientation therapy and related methods are usually not recommended by medical practitioners because they are often counter-productive to optimum care.

MYTH #10
Because someone in my family has or had Alzheimer's disease, I'm going to get it.

No, not necessarily. Having one first degree relative with Alzheimer's does not significantly increase the likelihood that you will get it. There are many factors that influence the possibility that someone will develop Alzheimer's disease, with genetics playing a role in fewer than seven percent of the cases. However, a person with two first degree relatives [such as a parent and a sibling or both parents] with Alzheimer's does have a higher risk but it is not a certain outcome. [2]

MYTH #11
Alzheimer's disease is a disease that only affects older people.

Unfortunately, that is not true as some people in mid-life develop Alzheimer's, frontotemporal, or other dementia diseases. These diseases are not a normal part of aging. [2]

Myth #12
Memory loss means Alzheimer's disease.

No, not necessarily. Many seniors have difficulty remembering various things, with names being one of the most common. But this does not mean they have developed Alzheimer's disease. When memory loss affects day-to-day activities especially when other functions such as lack of judgment, difficulty reasoning, and changes in communicational abilities occur, then it's best to consult a medical practitioner to evaluate the symptoms. [2]

MYTH # 13
Aluminum causes Alzheimer's disease.

No, this prevailing myth has never been substantiated. Most medical practitioners believe that the disease develops due to many combined risk factors. Age, genetics, lifestyle and environmental factors are believed to be the major culprits that team up to cause Alzheimer's. [2]

MYTH # 14
Alzheimer's disease is preventable.

No, that is not true. There is no single medication or combination of medications, lifestyle, diet, cognitive training, physical fitness exercises, stress reduction techniques or anything else that will prevent the onset of Alzheimer's. Rather, there is a combination of factors that can reduce the likelihood of developing Alzheimer's or delay its initiation. [2]

MYTH # 15
People with Alzheimer's disease cannot understand what is going on around them.

Wrong. It is true that the processing ability of a loved one living with Alzheimer's is much slower than formerly. It is also true that their communicational abilities are greatly reduced. However, they do understand much as they retain the ability to read body language and, given patience, they do understand much of what is said in one-on-one conversations. They just process conversations much more slowly than previously. The important point to remember is that a loved one living with Alzheimer's disease is still the same person they were previously but has a greater need to be treated with dignity and respect. [2]

What Worked for Us That May Work for You

- I accepted that dementia is just another serious disease like cancer, diabetes, heart and circulatory diseases.
- I learned as much as I could about dementia to prepare myself to deal with the future challenges.
- I found that empathetic listening and effective communication was the very best approach to help Laura.
- I listened to the medical advice furnished by our primary medical provider and found it of great value. Unfortunately, I was unable to utilize all of his referrals to various medical specialists due to Laura's strong opposition and belief that specialized tests and evaluations would be a waste of time.
- We took the primary medical provider prescribed drugs like statins, blood pressure reduction drugs, and bone density medications.

- We took approved supplements like a daily multivitamin and fish oil capsules.
- Following the Mediterranean diet and a Plant Based MIND Diet. The MIND diet is a special plant-based diet that combines the best features of the well-known Mediterranean diet with the lesser-known Dietary Approaches to Stop Hypertension (DASH) diet. MIND stands for the Mediterranean-DASH Intervention for Neurodegenerative Delay. [3]
- We consumed less than one tablespoon (about 14 grams) of unhealthy fats (saturated fats such as butter and margarine) daily. [3]

What Didn't Work for Us

- Reality Orientation therapy and related methods were counter-productive to optimum care after Laura progressed to the late moderate and severe stages. In the mild and early moderate stages, I used these methods with caution as Laura strongly opposed my overt attempts to use Reality Orientation as it was only marginally effective in her case.
- Internet or television medical infomercials giving free advice and asking you to purchase CD(s), DVD(s), book(s), magazine(s), newsletter(s) or product(s). I found that pursuing these options and alternatives were a waste of time and money.
- Consuming large amounts of healthy fats such as coconut oil.

Positive Affirmations

"There's no such thing as ruining your life. Life's a pretty resilient thing, it turns out." – *Sophie Kinsella*

"If you don't like something, change it. If you can't change it, change the way you think about it." – *Mary Engelbreit*

"Have courage for the great sorrows of life and patience for the small ones; and when you have laboriously accomplished your daily task, go to sleep in peace." – *Victor Hugo*

End Notes

[1]   https://www.ncbi.nim.nih.gov/pubmed/11034600

[2]   https://www.alzheimer.ca/sites/default/files/files/nation

[3]   https://www.healthline.com/nutrition/nubd-diet

CHAPTER 3

What is NOT Dementia

"My scars remind me that I did indeed survive my deepest wounds. That in itself is an accomplishment. And they bring to mind something else, too. They remind me that the damage life has inflicted on me has, in many places, left me stronger and more resilient. What hurt me in the past has actually made me better equipped to face the present."
– Steve Goodier

How did I know Laura's behavior was changing? Laura started to have cognitive, physical and emotional symptoms that baffled me. When I felt that I may become a future caregiver for Laura, my stress level increased. I felt a high personal concern that she could be entering dementia. Naturally, I had an associated high sense of urgency to determine if it was dementia. Anyone would feel the same. When Laura's personality changed and she started to show signs of problems and issues, questions ran through my mind like wildfire: Did Laura have dementia or was it something else? I hoped and prayed it was something else, and carefully researched the "something else" possibilities.

- Was it empty-nest syndrome?
- Could it be post-menopausal changes?
- Was it a vitamin or mineral deficiency?
- Was it due to our family members, friends and acquaintances being mean?

- Were Laura's signs simple senior moments?
- Could the signs be self-perceived by her as subjective cognitive impairment?
- Was it actual mild cognitive impairment?
- Could it possibly be some form of pseudodementia?

The ugly truth we experienced is this: Every person with dementia is different and has different progressions. Unfortunately, dementia symptoms cannot be resolved or cured but can be moderated and reduced when effective caregiving techniques are used. This is the main purpose of this book.

Senior Moments are not Dementia

Like everyone after a certain age, Laura had senior moments. I have senior moments. It is a non-medical term for mental glitches. Every senior I know has senior moments occasionally. Don't sweat the senior moments. From my observations, I believe senior moments occur more frequently to older seniors than younger seniors. But I have observed them to sometimes happen to younger and middle-aged adults also. Senior moments should be simply acknowledged, then corrected and/or apologized for, then forgotten/disregarded as a simple reality that occurs in the lives of most seniors.

Senior moments can occasionally include ...

- Forgetting names of people
- Cannot recall a telephone number of someone you call often
- Forgetting the PIN number associated with your debit card
- Drawing a blank when speaking and can't think of the correct word
- Being distracted while driving and missing the correct turn while traveling to a well-known destination
- Walking into a room to perform a task but forgetting the task
- Making mistakes involving judgment
- Becoming irritated or angered by a simple problem or issue

- Embarrassing yourself or others by saying the wrong word or using the wrong context
- Forgetting an important appointment
- Misplacing personal items such as car keys
- Cannot find reading glasses
- Having difficulty remembering recent conversations, what you have just read in the book or magazine, what you have just seen in a movie, television or live stage performance

Subjective Cognitive Impairment/ Decline is not Dementia

Subjective Cognitive Impairment/Decline is when people self-perceive they have worsening memory loss and other thinking inabilities. But this self-perception is separate and distinct from cognitive testing, clinical diagnosis or the observations of other people. Laura and I both had this self-observed concern. It's subjective because others did not have a perception that either of our thinking processes had declined. [1]

Laura felt it was not important whether she was or was not entering cognitive decline. I could never convince her to engage in cognitive testing, but I did so myself. When I did, I scored in the top ten percent compared to other males in my age group. When given this feedback, I commented that I felt sorry for the bottom 90 percent. I was told that I was personally too self-critical and too self-absorbed about the possibility that I had entered dementia.

Subjective Cognitive Impairment is also called subjective memory loss, subjective memory disorder, self-reported memory loss and subjective cognitive decline. [2] Not everyone who experiences the feeling of subjective cognitive decline eventually develops Mild Cognitive Impairment or a dementia disease, but some do. The Behavioral Risk Factor Surveillance System (BRFSS) survey, which included questions on self-perceived confusion and memory loss, found that in 2015-2016, 11% of Americans aged 45 and older reported subjective cognitive decline, but 55% of those who reported it had not consulted a health care professional about it. [2] So, it appears that Laura and I almost exactly match the outcome of this survey.

In summary, subjective cognitive impairment/decline is not dementia. As part of my feedback when I had cognitive testing, I remember being told that a person should not look too hard to find something, because if you look hard enough, you may eventually find it.

Mild Cognitive Impairment (MCI) is not Dementia

There is a gray area between the senior moments of normal aging and mild dementia. It is called Mild Cognitive Impairment or MCI.

Laura had MCI for several years. Since we were so close, I recognized it since her memory, reasoning and judgment declined when compared to the former prime years of her life.

MCI symptoms are not harmful and are easily recognized by a spouse or a child with whom you have close daily contact. Realizing that a loved one has MCI is important as it presents daily challenges for both the loved one and the caregiver. Since the challenges are relatively minor, it is important to simply accept the new reality and deal with it in a positive manner.

The word "cognitive" is probably not in your everyday vocabulary. It is a somewhat technical term that serves like an umbrella word that has many meanings. It includes the processes of thinking, remembering, reasoning, computing, speaking, listening, understanding, learning, knowing, perceiving and judging. The medical profession uses cognitive as a somewhat ambiguous or general term. Caregivers must adapt and learn to use it also.

MCI may or may not be diagnosed by a loved one's personal medical provider. If it is, then it may be the first warning that dementia may follow. About one-quarter of the people diagnosed with MCI will progress into mild dementia in about five years. Roughly another quarter will have mild dementia in ten years while one-half will remain relatively stable and live with MCI symptoms for the remainder of their lives. Some people diagnosed with MCI may improve. Many seniors have symptoms of MCI but are able to live independently. Due to the complexity of the brain, these changes vary between individuals and are often difficult to recognize. Since these changes do not significantly interfere with a person's life, they are typically ignored by the senior.

The difference between normal senior moments and MCI is the frequency of the occurrences. Senior moments seldom or less occasionally occur while MCI issues occur more often.

Often, MCI symptoms include:

- Often forgetting names of people
- Often forgetting a telephone number of someone you call often
- Often forgetting the PIN number associated with your debit card
- Often drawing a blank when speaking and can't think of the correct word
- Often being distracted while driving and missing the correct turn while traveling to a well-known destination
- Often walking into a room to perform a task, but forgetting the task
- Often making mistakes involving judgment
- Often becoming irritated or angered by a simple problem or issue
- Often making mistakes or embarrassing yourself or others by saying the wrong word or using the wrong context
- Often forgetting an important appointment
- Often misplacing personal items such as car keys
- Often cannot fine reading glasses
- Often having difficulty remembering recent conversations
- Often having difficulty remembering what you have just read in the book or magazine, or what you have just seen in a movie, television or live stage performance

Yes, these are identical to senior moment symptoms but the critical difference is that senior moment symptoms are occasional occurrences and MCI symptoms happen with more regularity.

Recovering from Surgery is not Dementia

When seniors enter a hospital for a medical procedure requiring general anesthesia, they may wind up with memory and/or cognitive defects for days or weeks following surgery. For most, it is completely resolved within a few months.

Pseudodementia is not Dementia

Here is a handy table of dementia and pseudodementia symptoms. Pseudodementia is defined by Wikipedia as a condition whose presenting symptoms appear as dementia, but actually result from depression or the side effects of medications being taken.

DEMENTIA	PSEUDODEMENTIA
Loses interest in hobbies and formerly pleasurable activities very slowly over several years	Loses interest in hobbies and formerly pleasurable activities in weeks or months
Someone with true dementia usually does not express anxiety and is often unconcerned about any cognitive loss issues. That person will minimize any loss of cognitive abilities and will minimize, rationalize and usually deny having any issues. The progression of true dementia takes years.	This person often appears worried and distressed. The onset of pseudodementia occurs in a matter of weeks. He or she may express anxiety and fear of losing their mind, will exaggerate his or her fears of having cognitive defects and be preoccupied with concentration and focus issues.
The loved one living with dementia experiences something called "sundowning" which is a general term when a person has anxiety and agitation in the evening.	A loved one with pseudodementia and depression has anxiety and agitation early in the morning.

DEMENTIA	PSEUDODEMENTIA
It's common for the person living with dementia to have anxiety and agitation in new environments and new situations.	The person with depression can meet new environments and situations without anxiety and agitation being experienced.
The loved one living with dementia will rarely be suicidal, feel guilty or feel worthless.	A loved one with pseudodementia with severe depression may be suicidal, feel a strong sense of guilt and feel worthless.
When tested and evaluated, the loved one living with dementia is usually inattentive and has greater impairment of short term rather than long-term memory. That person may cooperate with testing and try to guess or bluff his or her answers during testing.	When tested and evaluated, the person suffering with pseudodementia is usually attentive, but will complain of both kinds of memory loss. They will be often uncooperative, insisting that he or she cannot pass any memory test. However, when tested, he or she will perform better than what they describe.
When the person living with dementia is treated for depression, the results rarely result in a full reversal of the cognitive impairments.	When depression is treated, the person with pseudodementia often responds positively.

What Worked for Us That May Work for You

- Make it a habit to do one thing at a time, i.e. avoid multi-tasking
- Learn and use stress management techniques like deep breathing, progressive relaxation and meditation
- Keep personal items in the same location

- Keep a calendar with important appointments clearly entered
- Review the calendar each morning and then make a to-do list of what should be accomplished each day
- Make periodic notes of items needed from stores
- Form a habit to be 15 minutes early for appointments and use the extra time to relax, socialize or meditate
- Handle mail each day when it arrives. Immediately place junk mail into your recycling container
- Keep check-off lists of periodic bills and recurring expenses
- Discard or donate unused items
- Make it a priority to avoid physical and mental clutter
- You can only keep one thought in your mind at a time. Replace negative thoughts with positive affirmations
- Make it a habit to remember names of persons you have just met by forming a mental image of an easily remembered visual and associating it with that person
- Make it a habit to be more observant. Notice how things look, smell, taste and feel. Notice what is happening in the environment at the time you make the observation. Try to remember things in multiple ways with connections to helpful details
- When reading, watching a movie, television or live performance, form a habit of occasionally taking a time-out or break to review and summarize the content of what you have just received
- Learn memory tricks such as mnemonic abbreviations, e.g. ROY G BIV [red, orange, yellow, green, blue, indigo and violet] for the colors in the spectrum
- Replay important memories in your mind to better reinforce their details
- Relax. Senior moments and Subjective Cognitive Impairment/ Decline thoughts are relatively harmless. Knowing they occur and dealing with them is a normal occurrence for most seniors.

Positive Affirmations

"Whether you think you can or can't, either way you are right." – *Megan Street*

"The best people possess a feeling for beauty, the courage to take risks, the discipline to tell the truth, the capacity for sacrifice. Ironically, their virtues make them vulnerable; they are often wounded, sometimes destroyed." – *Ernest Hemingway*

"Happiness is an attitude. We either make ourselves miserable or happy and strong. The amount of work is the same." – *Francesca Reigler*

"Our greatest glory is not in never falling, but in rising every time we fall." – *Confucius*

"Problems are not stop signs; they are guidelines." – *Robert Schuller*

"We must meet the challenge rather than wish it were not before us." – *William J. Brennan, Jr.*

End Notes

[1]   https://www.alz.org/media/Documents/alzheimers-facts-and-figures-2019

[2]   https://www.verywellhealth.com/subjective-cognitive-impairment

CHAPTER 4

What Exactly is Dementia?

*"Kindness can transform someone's dark moment with a
blaze of light. You'll never know how much your caring
matters. Make a difference for another day."*
– Amy Leigh Mercree

Dementia is scary, but it is not the name of a specific disease. Dementia is an umbrella word or general term for a group of symptoms and these symptoms are primarily cognitive disorders. Just like the word automobile doesn't describe individual makes or models and the word vegetable doesn't describe the many specific types of this food source, dementia doesn't uniquely describe any specific disease. It summarizes the types of symptoms that occur in several types of dementia.

The most common diagnosis of dementia is Alzheimer's disease, followed by Vascular dementia, mixed dementia (both Alzheimer's and Vascular together), Lewy Body dementia, Frontotemporal dementia, Parkinson's Disease dementia and others. There are more than 50 dementia diseases in all according to some sources. [1]

All of the dementia diseases are progressive diseases. This means that the structure and chemistry of the brain neurons and their associated connections deteriorate slowly and gradually over time. Some practitioners refer to dementia as brain failure similar to heart failure, kidney failure or other organ failure. Laura's ability to think gradually declined including her ability to remember, communicate, reason and understand.

Laura had progressive neurodegenerative brain disease caused by Alzheimer's, vascular disease, and Lewy Body disease with a diagnosis of mixed dementia. When a decline in memory function is severe enough to interfere with daily life, it is called dementia. Unfortunately, there is no cure for dementia and there is nothing that will slow its progression. The loved one who is impacted will have a reduced life span. However, the degree of the severity of the symptoms and the quality of life of the loved one with dementia can be significantly improved through effective caregiver actions.

There is a well-known statement which accurately describes the disease:

**If you know one person with dementia,
you know one person with dementia.**

The reason this is so often quoted is because of the unique differences and complexities of dementia. Although no two people with dementia have an identical progression, most experience the three main stages: Mild, moderate and severe. How you best deal with each stage is to be prepared and armed with coping strategies by knowing specifics of the progression and symptoms of each stage.

In the mild stage, Laura and I traveled frequently to Western Europe and throughout the United States. In the early moderate stage, we only traveled with assistance from another couple. Later in the moderate stage, we only travel within a day's drive from our home. And in the severe stage, we did not leave our city.

Stage Duration

There is no set length of time any person living with dementia will stay in any particular stage. Each one can last a few years or could be more than a decade. The progression through the stages is also unique for every individual. Why? In my research I've found that every human brain is so extremely complex that no other possibility exists.

Which stage was Laura in the longest? It was the mild stage which lasted over a decade. What applies to one person does not always apply to others. The type of dementia, the age the dementia begins, other illnesses, the loved one's environment, the level of person-centered care, knowledgeable support and other factors uniquely impact each individual's quality and length of life.

Some maintain their independence for many years. In the middle and later stages of dementia, they will need more and more support with daily activities like cooking or personal care such as washing and dressing. While dementia shortens life expectancy, some people live with it for many years.

Other Things to Keep in Mind

Overlap

Overlap can occur between the stages. For example, some handle an activity well in the mild or moderate stage yet others have difficulty with the same activity while in the mild stage. What does this mean? Your loved one may need assistance with one specific task but be able to handle others on their own.

No Linear Progression

Dementia is fickle. There is no exact linear progression of the dementia stages. Some symptoms may appear in the mild stage in some people or be delayed or non-existent in others. Some symptoms may seem to improve and others may switch back and forth between stages randomly.

Simultaneous Stages / Worsening Symptoms

It's also possible that your loved one may appear as though he or she is in two progressive stages simultaneously. Laura had visual perception issues early in the mild stage but others may not experience visual perception difficulties until much later.

And then you may find that some symptoms will appear, worsen and then gradually disappear. There was a severe stage period when Laura became loud, verbally aggressive and used vulgar language. Later, she reverted to her normal sweet, soft-spoken, kind self.

Wandering

Some people wander in the moderate stage, and never wander after they enter the severe stage. Others do not begin to wander until the severe stage. Laura had a potential for wandering in both the moderate and severe stages but, fortunately, it was rare when she wandered outside. That was a very important blessing as wandering outside can be extremely dangerous.

What Worked for Us That May Work for You

- Although dementia cannot be currently cured or slowed, the symptoms can be moderated. How? Simply by following well-known medical advice.
- What is good for your loved one's heart is good for their brain. The brain is a small percentage of a person's weight but uses 20 percent of the blood pumped by the heart.
- Annual or semi-annual routine visits to a primary care physician.
- Heart and stroke preventive lifestyles.
- Physical exercise.
- Diet: Vegan, plant based, Mediterranean and MIND diets are all good.
- No nicotine consumption, alcohol consumption or mind-altering drug consumption in any form.
- A good night's sleep including sleep apnea control, if needed.
- Learning new facts, skills, games and procedures.
- Socialization with close family and friends as well as with strangers.
- Participating in board games of any kind, such as bingo or card games.

- Being an active member of an organized club, religious or volunteer group.

Positive Affirmations

"No matter what you've done for yourself or for humanity, if you can't look back on having given love and attention to your own family, what have you really accomplished." – *Lee Iacocca*

End Note

[1]   https://www.webmd.com/alzheimers/types-dementia

CHAPTER 5

What Exactly is Alzheimer's Disease?

"I am not sure exactly what heaven will be like, but I do know that when we die and it comes time for God to judge us, He will not ask, 'How many good things have you done in your life?,' rather He will ask, 'How much love did you put into what you did?'"
– Mother Theresa

Alzheimer's disease is a riddle hidden inside an enigma only to be understood by a genius who can solve a Rubik's Cube in less than three seconds. This is not an exaggeration. I believe this is an actual understatement of the complexities of this disease. Here's how Alzheimer's Weekly describes it:

> "Alzheimer's disease is a major unsolved puzzle in medical research. Currently, there is no cure, no effective treatment, not even certainty about its cause. As Alzheimer's disease progresses, brain tissue shrinks and dies. This causes a gradual loss of short-term memory, difficulties thinking, confusion and behavioral changes, ultimately leading to death." [1]

As stated in previous chapters, Laura had Alzheimer's disease based on her progression. Additionally, she had vascular dementia based on brain scans and, to complicate matters, she had

Lewy Body dementia based on her history of delusions, hallucinations and visual-spatial issues. Due to the complexity of accurately diagnosing a specific dementia disease, Laura and many
others living with dementia receive the catch-all diagnosis of
mixed dementia.

Alzheimer's Disease

Alzheimer's disease symptoms are known to overlap other dementia diseases. So, a quick review or summary is always useful. The
U.S. Alzheimer's Association has published the 10 warning signs of
Alzheimer's disease and other similar organizations world-wide
publish almost identical information. The following well-written
table is an exact quote from the online summaries of Alzheimer's
organizations in the U.S., England, Wales, Northern Ireland and
Australia. Similar summaries appear in Alzheimer's organizations
in Scotland, Canada, Europe, Asia and Latin America. [1, 2, 3]

Alzheimer's Symptoms	Age-Related Symptoms
Memory loss that disrupts daily life: One of the most common signs of Alzheimer's is memory loss, especially forgetting recently learned information. Others include forgetting important dates or events, asking for the same information over and over and increasingly needing to rely on memory aids like reminder notes or electronic devices or family members for things that used to be handled on one's own.	Sometimes forgetting names or appointments but remembering them later.

Alzheimer's Symptoms	Age-Related Symptoms
Challenges in planning or solving problems: Some people experience changes in their ability to develop and follow a plan or work with numbers. They may have trouble following a familiar recipe, keeping track of monthly bills or counting change. They may have difficulty concentrating and take much longer to do things than they did before.	Making occasional errors when balancing a checkbook.
Difficulty completing familiar tasks at home, at work or at leisure: People with Alzheimer's often find it hard to complete daily tasks. Sometimes, people have trouble driving to a familiar location, managing a budget at work or remembering the rules of a favorite game.	Occasionally needing help to use the settings on a microwave or to record a television show.
Confusion with time or place: People with Alzheimer's can lose track of dates, seasons and the passage of time. They may have trouble understanding something if it is not happening immediately. Sometimes they forget where they are or how they got there.	Getting confused about the day of the week but figuring it out later.

Alzheimer's Symptoms	Age-Related Symptoms
Trouble understanding visual images and spatial relationships: For some people, having vision problems is a sign of Alzheimer's. They may have difficulty reading, judging distance and determining color or contrast which may cause problems with driving.	Vision changes related to cataracts.
New problems with words in speaking or writing: People with Alzheimer's may have trouble following or joining a conversation. They may stop in the middle of a conversation and have no idea how to continue or they may repeat themselves. They may struggle with vocabulary, have problems finding the right word or call things by the wrong name (e.g., calling a watch a hand clock).	Sometimes having trouble finding the right word.
Misplacing things and losing the ability to retrace steps: People with Alzheimer's may put things in unusual places and lose things and be unable to go back over their steps to find them again. Sometimes, they accuse others of stealing. This may occur more frequently over time.	Misplacing things from time to time and retracing steps to find them.

Alzheimer's Symptoms	Age-Related Symptoms
Decreased or poor judgment: People with Alzheimer's may experience changes in judgment or decision making. For example, they may use poor judgment when dealing with money, giving large amounts to telemarketers. They may pay less attention to grooming or keeping themselves clean.	Making a bad decision once in a while.
Withdrawal from work or social activities: People with Alzheimer's may start to remove themselves from hobbies, social activities, work projects or sports. They may have trouble keeping up with a favorite sports team or remembering how to complete a favorite hobby. They may also avoid being social because of the changes they have experienced.	Sometimes feeling weary of work, family and social obligations.
Changes in mood and personality: The mood and personalities of people with Alzheimer's can change. They can become confused, suspicious, depressed, fearful or anxious. They may be easily upset at home, at work, with friends or in places where they are out of their comfort zones.	Developing very specific ways of doing things and becoming irritable when a routine is disrupted.

Severe Dementia

Why is severe dementia called Alzheimer's disease? Because in 1907, psychiatrist and physician Alois Alzheimer studied a patient with severe dementia until the patient died. Following death, Alzheimer autopsied the body including the patient's brain. He found plaques and tangles in the shrunken and diseased brain and documented his findings in a report filed with the German patent office. Later, he presented his findings in a medical conference held in Munich, Germany. [4]

Paralleling Alzheimer's work, Oskar Fischer worked in the German Hospital and University of Prague (then part of Austria-Hungary) in the same year, 1907. Fischer studied numerous patients with severe dementia and, following their deaths, autopsied their bodies and brains. He found plaques and tangles in the brains of 16 individuals and documented his findings in a report also filed with the German patent office. [5]

Oskar Fischer is actually the co-founder of Alzheimer's disease. How much of Fischer's information was known to Alzheimer? How much of Alzheimer's information was known to Fischer? It is not clear, but perhaps all of it. Why isn't this disease called either Alzheimer-Fischer Disease or Fischer-Alzheimer Disease? Politics is the answer as Alzheimer had a better mentor. This mentor had tremendous political skills, high status and wide connections. Also, the Munich scientific community happened to be dominant during that era. Naturally, there was serious competition for funding between the Munich Hospital and University and the German Hospital and University in Prague. These factors resulted in Alzheimer's research being recognized world-wide for over 100 years and Alzheimer became famous for it.

Fischer's extensive research findings, reports and expertise were buried in the medical archives in Prague only to be discovered and published in 2008. Some medical experts, researchers and scientists currently believe that Fischer's work was so advanced that it was the best available in 1907 and far better than Alzheimer's. [6]

Enough history. Let's look at what Alzheimer's disease is and what you should look for.

Hallmarks of Alzheimer's

The hallmarks of Alzheimer's involve problems with language, such as finding the right word for something. I'm not talking about the odd occasion when we all are at a loss for the right word. This is much more serious than that.

The loved one with Alzheimer's feels confused or finds it hard to follow what is being said. He or she also has problems with seeing objects in three dimensions, difficulty with everyday activities like getting confused with coins when paying for items at a store, becoming more withdrawn and experiencing mood swings.

The Alzheimer's Association estimates that more than five million people in the United States of all ages are living with Alzheimer's disease. This organization advises that it is the sixth-leading cause of death in the U.S. and is the only top 10 cause of death that cannot be prevented, cured or even slowed. [7]

Alzheimer's disease is thought to start making brain changes 20 years or more before symptoms begin. A healthy human brain has about 100 billion neurons each with long branching extensions to other neurons. These neuron to neuron connections are called synapses and there are roughly 100 trillion of them or about 1,000 connections per neuron. Signals go through these synapses to and from neurons to provide memories, thoughts, sensations, emotions, movements and skills. [4] The disease attacks these connections but the enormous size and complexity of the brain circuits compensates for the cells killed by the disease during those 20 or so years.

What Causes Alzheimer's Disease

An incontrovertible diagnosis of Alzheimer's disease (versus probable Alzheimer's disease) cannot be conclusively made while a person is living. However, after the person dies and a neuropathologist examines brain tissue sample under a microscope and finds beta amyloid plaques and tau tangles (the abnormal proteins that are believed to confirm Alzheimer's disease), a definitive diagnosis can be made.

This statement assumes, however, that the current scientific belief that amyloid plaques (sticky microscopic clumps of stray amyloid proteins that form outside the brain cell) and tau protein tangles (abnormally twisted fibers of tau protein that form inside the brain cell) are the actual causes of this disease.

Disagreement Among Scientists

Some researchers believe the beta amyloid plaques are the cause, but others believe the tau protein tangles are responsible. Still, other researchers take the middle ground and support both theories. And then there are some researchers who believe that some other factor is the cause such as a brain infection.

Another possibility is called type 3 diabetes. It is fairly well-known that late adult onset (type 2) diabetes may cause up to a 60 percent increase in the instance of Alzheimer's disease. This may be due to a combination of several factors. Diabetes causes damage to the blood vessels in the brain (a hallmark of vascular dementia), increased inflammation in the brain (triggered by high blood sugar levels) and a disruption of the chemicals in the brain impacts the balance of the brain chemicals used for communication between brain neurons. The science of this is still shaky.

Some scientists believe the cause of Alzheimer's disease is currently unknown. Why? Because the researchers who conduct autopsies after death and examine brain tissue of some perfectly cognizant seniors, often find the same characteristic plaques and tangles. These findings prompt many researchers to believe that some other condition may be the actual cause.

Naturally, this complicates the forward motion of research as tremendous efforts are currently being made world-wide to find ways to reduce beta amyloid plaques and tau protein tangles in the brains of laboratory mice and, therefore, to eventually do so in the human brain.

What's the tripwire when it comes to finding a definitive cause? Autopsies by neuropathologists are expensive and, therefore, not common; so, a clear conclusion is not possible right now which handicaps researchers in the quest for a cure.

Mice Experimentation

Laboratory studies have introduced both the beta amyloid plaques and tau tangles into the brains of mice and gave them dementia. Later, they cured them. So, the researchers seem to be able to cure dementia in mice but not in humans at this time and, sadly, many major pharmaceutical companies have abandoned their search for a cure.

I apologize if this information makes any caregiver lose hope for a cure. The above discussion is provided to augment my opening paragraph on the complexity of the disease and the human brain.

There is always hope as numerous world-wide initiatives are being addressed. This information is provided only as a reality check and to encourage you, as a caregiver, to strive for your best efforts each day and maintain your focus on ways to improve the quality of life for your loved one.

For Laura and me, it didn't really matter what name was given to describe severe dementia. In the severe stage, almost all dementias have similar symptoms. The name Alzheimer's disease is commonly used worldwide and is generally clearly understood. However, in this book I will use the term dementia to include Alzheimer's disease and also encompass numerous other progressive neurodegenerative diseases.

What Worked for Us That May Work for You

As a caregiver, I accepted that the lack of progress in the past one hundred years will probably continue. I strove to maintain my focus on the quality of care and the quality of life for Laura. I did my best to give her the TLC she deserved.

Positive Affirmations

"Some days there won't be a song in your heart. Sing anyway." – *Emory Austin*

"Forgiveness is not an occasional act; it is a constant attitude." – *Martin Luther King Jr.*

End Notes

[1]   https://www.alz.org/media/Documents/alzheimers-facts-and-figures-2019-r.pdf

[2]   https://www.alz.org/uk/dementia-alzheimers-uk

[3]   https://www.alz.org/au/dementia-alzheimers-au

[4]   alzheimersweekly.com/2015/02

[5]   https://www.alzheimer.neurology.ucla.edu

[6]   htttps://www.ncbi.nim.nih.gov/pmd/articles/PMC2

[7]   https://www.alz.org/media/Documents/alzheimers-facts-and-figures-2019-r.pdf

CHAPTER 6

What are Some Other Dementia Diseases?

"You have to accept whatever comes and the only important thing is that you meet it with courage and with the best that you have to give."
– Eleanor Roosevelt

When a caregiver suspects his or her loved one is living with mild dementia, several questions arise:

- Is it dementia?
- If so, what type is it?

Laura had mixed dementia and the exact types are difficult for a caregiver to recognize. In fact, it may be so difficult to recognize that it is probably impossible for a layperson serving as a caregiver to recognize the exact type(s). Knowing the early symptoms of each type can be enormously beneficial in making certain caregiving decisions.

We've already covered the symptoms of Alzheimer's in the previous chapter. Here are some other dementia diseases to watch out for:

- Vascular
- Parkinson's
- Lewy Body

- Frontotemporal
- Progressive Supranuclear Palsy, and
- Mixed

Reference numbers for information relating to each of the diseases come at the end of each section.

Vascular Disease Dementia

In early stages, this condition causes the loved one living with dementia to experience cognitive difficulty with reasoning and judgment. Common early changes include difficulty planning, thinking quickly or concentrating. There might also be short periods when he or she gets very confused. The loved one may also become depressed or anxious. However, memory loss isn't always common in the early stages.

If the loved one has a severe stroke, symptoms of vascular dementia can begin suddenly. He or she can then remain stable or, in the early stages, might even get a little bit better over time. If he or she then has another stroke, the symptoms might worsen.

If the loved one has a series of less severe strokes, his or her symptoms may remain stable for a while and then get worse in stages rather than experiencing a gradual decline. Vascular dementia can also result if the loved one has other conditions that damage blood vessels and reduce circulation. These conditions include the wear and tear of blood vessels due to aging, high blood pressure, atherosclerosis, diabetes and brain hemorrhage.

Vascular disease dementia symptoms often overlap with those of other types of dementia, especially Alzheimer's disease dementia. Vascular dementia signs and symptoms include:

1. Confusion
2. Trouble paying attention and concentrating
3. Reduced ability to organize thoughts or actions
4. Decline in ability to analyze a situation, develop an effective action plan and communicate that plan to others

5. Difficulty deciding what to do next
6. Restlessness and agitation
7. Unsteady gait
8. Sudden or frequent urge to urinate or inability to control passing urine
9. Depression or apathy [1]

Parkinson's Disease Dementia:
Parkinson's disease is an age-related degenerative disorder of certain brain cells. Parkinson's often starts with a tremor in one hand and those tremors increase to include both hands, arms, jaw and face. The hallmark of this disease involves physical movement issues including slow and rigid movements, stiffness and loss of balance and coordination. The loved one also has disturbed sleep patterns and gradual cognitive deterioration. Slowness of movement, shuffling, speaking very softly and presenting an expressionless face are all common symptoms. At the final stages of Parkinson's disease, the dementia symptoms often become apparent.

Parkinson's disease dementia signs and symptoms include:

1. Changes in memory, concentration and judgment
2. Trouble interpreting visual information
3. Muffled speech
4. Visual hallucinations
5. Delusions, especially paranoid ideas
6. Depression
7. Irritability and anxiety
8. Sleep disturbances, including excessive daytime drowsiness and rapid eye movement (REM) sleep disorder. [2]

Lewy Body Dementia

Most experts estimate that Lewy Body dementia is the third most common cause of dementia after Alzheimer's disease and Vascular disease dementias. It accounts for five to ten percent of the cases of dementia. The hallmark brain abnormalities are called Lewy bodies and named after Frederich H. Lewy, M.D., the neurologist who discovered them while working for Dr. Alois Alzheimer in the early 1900s.

In the early stages of dementia with Lewy bodies, the loved one might find it hard to stay alert and have difficulty with planning ahead, reasoning and solving problems. These symptoms typically vary a lot from one day to the next.

He or she might also have problems with vision, such as finding it hard to judge distances, problems with seeing objects in three dimensions or seeing things that aren't really there (visual hallucinations).

Lewy Body seems to be a first cousin to Parkinson's Disease. The loved one may or may not develop symptoms like those in Parkinson's disease, but if they do, they would include slow and rigid movements, problems balancing and trembling of an arm or leg.

Disturbed sleep patterns are also common. However, the loved one's memory will often be affected less than in someone with Alzheimer's disease. Note that some types of antipsychotics are extremely dangerous to those with Lewy Body dementia.

Lewy Body dementia signs and symptoms include:

1. Changes in thinking and reasoning
2. Confusion and alertness that varies significantly from one time of day to another or from one day to the next
3. Slowness, gait imbalance and other Parkinsonian movement features
4. Well-formed visual hallucinations
5. Delusions
6. Trouble interpreting visual information
7. Sleep disturbance
8. Malfunctions of the automatic (autonomic) nervous system
9. Memory loss that may be significant but less prominent than in Alzheimer's [3]

Frontotemporal Disease Dementia

The symptoms of FTD involve deterioration of decision-making, behavioral control, emotional control and language skills. Behavior, personality, language and movement are affected. The drugs given to people with Alzheimer's haven't been shown to offer any benefits to people with frontotemporal dementia and they may even be harmful. The loved one's personal physician must make an individual decision in this case.

If a person has behavioral variant frontotemporal dementia, it's common to be prescribed antidepressant medication. This can reduce inappropriate and obsessive or compulsive behaviors.

Frontotemporal disease dementia signs and symptoms include:

1. Poor judgment
2. Loss of empathy
3. Socially inappropriate behavior
4. Lack of inhibition
5. Repetitive compulsive behavior
6. Inability to concentrate or plan
7. Frequent, abrupt mood changes
8. Speech difficulties [4]

Progressive Supranuclear Palsy Dementia

In the early stages of Progressive Supranuclear Palsy (PSP), the loved one has serious and progressive problems with walking, gait and balance as well as eye movement and thinking problems. Falling over backward is common with PSP. It is not Parkinson's disease, but it is a Parkinsonian-like syndrome. It is also called Steele-Richardson-Olszewski syndrome.

Progressive supranuclear palsy (PSP) disease dementia signs and symptoms include:

1. Stiffness and awkward movements
2. Falling

3. Problems with speech and swallowing
4. Sensitivity to light
5. Sleep disturbances
6. Loss of interest in pleasurable activities
7. Impulsive behavior, possibly including laughing or crying for no reason
8. Difficulties with memory, reasoning, problem-solving and decision-making
9. Depression and anxiety
10. A surprised or frightened facial expression, resulting from rigid facial muscles [5]

Mixed Dementia

Laura was eventually diagnosed with mixed dementia, as she had clear evidence of Alzheimer's disease dementia based on her history, vascular dementia disease based on her brain scans and Lewy Body disease dementia based on her hallucinations, delusions and visual-spatial difficulties.

What Worked for Us That May Work for You

- Accepting that a precise diagnosis is extremely difficult
- Realizing that, as dementia progresses to the severe stage, the symptoms and the activities of daily living that are impacted are the same for everyone living with dementia

Positive Affirmations

"When you can think of yesterday without regret and tomorrow without fear, you are near contentment."
– *Unknown*

"Physical strength is measured by what we can carry; spiritual by what we can bear." – *Unknown*

"Certain defects are necessary for the existence of individu-ality." – *Johann Wolfgang von Goethe*

End Notes

[1]   https://www.mayoclinic.org/diseases-conditions/vasculardementia

[2]   https://www.emedicinehealth.com/parkinson_disease

[3]   https://www.alz.org/alzheimers-dementia/what-is-lewybody

[4]   https://www.mayoclinic.org/diseases-conditions/frontotemporaldementia

[5]   https://www.mayoclinic.org/diseases-conditions/progressivesupranuclearpalsydementia

CHAPTER 7

Cognitive (Communicational Types) Early Warning Signs

*"Never believe that a few caring people can't change
the world. For, indeed, that's all who ever have."*
– Margaret Mead, Anthropologist

The Signs of Dementia

The signs of dementia can be grouped into three areas: Cognitive, physical and emotional. These are the groupings I believe are the simplest to understand.

The cognitive symptoms can be grouped into many different categories, but for ease of understanding, I believe they are best grouped into three: The communicational type cognitive symptoms, the less complex type cognitive symptoms and the more complex type cognitive symptoms. The communicational type symptoms are usually the easiest to recognize, because verbal interactions are so basic.

The signs of dementia are important because medical specialists diagnose various different types of dementias based on their knowledge of different symptoms. However, I believe a medical dementia diagnosis is an inexact science.

The early warning signs and symptoms come in many different forms and, while some of them are easily recognizable, others can slip by unnoticed. Unfortunately, there is no absolute set or concrete pattern of symptoms to inform a caregiver at which stage and what specific form of dementia the loved one has.

Naturally, cognitive and communication symptoms overlap as do cognitive and physical symptoms as well as those attributed to cognitive and emotional. However, for purposes of describing them and for practical understanding how best the caregiver can deal with them, I summarize them into these three categories.

Laura's verbal communication issues were very subtle early in the mild stage. She effectively used her intelligence to compensate for speaking and listening deficiencies. In social situations and in normal nonspecific conversation, Laura did very well and it was almost impossible for others to recognize anything was wrong.

Laura's Challenges

By the end of the mild stage, Laura began to communicate poorly during shopping trips, in social interactions and at home. She had difficulty organizing her thoughts and expressing them, where previously she was highly social and verbal.

Laura's reading and writing skills slowly deteriorated. She could no longer write short thank you notes, which previously had been her custom. Laura no longer looked forward to the next publication of her favorite romance genre author. She no longer devoured our local newspaper early in the morning as she enjoyed her morning coffee.

Here are lists of some symptoms your loved one may experience.

General speaking difficulties:

- Sometimes a loss of words occurs when speaking
- Randomly finding it difficult to communicate clearly and effectively
- Every now and then, memory lapses occur finding it difficult to speak clearly and effectively
- Occasionally experiencing word-finding pauses when speaking

- Erratically experiencing brain fog and senior moments when speaking
- Beginning to struggle to communicate effectively using spoken words to communicate thoughts
- At times, being reluctant to make mistakes when speaking so avoiding speaking unless it is urgent

Starting to use vague, non-specific or incorrect spoken words:

- Randomly finding that it is difficult to find the right word for the specific context being discussed
- At times, having trouble or difficulty remembering the specific name of a person, place or thing
- Every now and then using vague or non-specific language
- From time to time, the ability to remember and properly use the exact meaning of words deteriorates
- Beginning to use substitute or generic words when the correct or appropriate word cannot be found, e.g., "the thing" instead of "the envelope"
- Sporadically making up nonsense words which are close in sound to the word intended to be said
- Occasionally using novel or invented words, making speech difficult to understand
- Sometimes using broad categories (the worker) when describing something instead of the specific noun or precise, descriptive word (the electrician)
- Beginning to use pronouns (he or she) instead of the specific name (Michael or Sherri)
- At times, saying the name of the whole object when a part of the object would be much more descriptive, e.g. "the tickets to the theater were in the coat" instead of "the tickets to the theater were in the inside breast pocket of the sports coat"
- Erratically having difficulty or trouble remembering or finding the correct or appropriate word for the thought being expressed

Unusual repetitions begin:

- Infrequently repeating the same question, phrase, story, or information several times within a few minutes or several times per day
- Sometimes repeating the same point several times, over and over again, in conversation

Listening difficulty occurs:

- Sporadically having difficulty understanding the meaning, idea or concept being expressed by another
- Sometimes not being able to follow verbal instructions
- From time to time, not able to understand and remember the exact or precise meaning of words
- Every now and then, not remembering names when meeting new people
- From time to time, having difficulty remembering what was just spoken to you
- At times, having trouble remembering the plot line and/or names of the famous actors or actresses of a movie or stage show just viewed
- Sometimes having trouble remembering the name of a famous news commentator just after he or she introduced himself or herself on television as the news show starts
- Occasionally, mentally drifting off and missing the entire thrust of a verbal message

Difficulty conversing begins:

- At times, having difficulty engaging in social conversation
- Occasionally, completely losing the thread of a conversation
- At times, being unable to understand the logic of moderately complex sentences

- From time to time, having trouble carrying on a conversation
- Sometimes struggling to follow a conversation or misinterpreting things heard
- Beginning to use the telephone less and saying less in phone conversations
- At times, having difficulty understanding the meaning, idea or concept being expressed by another
- Once in a while, having trouble or difficulty understanding and following a conversation with one person or among several people
- Occasionally avoiding casual conversations due to difficulty understanding
- From time to time, having difficulty remembering what was just spoken by you or to you
- Occasionally, relying on others to answer simple questions
- Every so often, becoming confused when speaking, especially when corrected by others
- Sometimes becoming distracted and finding it difficult to keep the conversation on the same subject
- Once in a while, becoming reluctant to make mistakes when speaking, so avoiding speaking unless it is urgent

Reading difficulties begin:

- At times, having less interest in reading the daily newspaper
- Having less interest in the pleasure reading of novels
- Occasionally, experiencing brain fog and senior moments when reading
- From time to time, when reading, the written content is difficult to understand
- Occasionally having trouble or difficulty remembering the main and/or minor points of what was just read in a book, magazine, newspaper or on a computer screen
- Occasionally asking someone else to read out loud the

personal notes from family and friends on Christmas and birthday cards

Writing difficulties occur:

- Sometimes the content being written is unclear and difficult to understand
- Sporadically having difficulty writing a thank you note
- Occasionally experiencing brain fog and senior moments when writing
- At times, the ability to generate written communications is degraded
- Every now and then, the cursive signature on credit cards is almost illegible

What Worked for Us That May Work for You

- Attempt to monitor visitors and social situations to control situations where the loved one is one-on-one with others when communicating
- Gradually inform and educate family members, neighbors and social contacts to keep conversations simple and avoid multiple questions in conversations
- Form the habit of summarizing useful information in the media to keep your loved one informed
- Purchase a telephone with large buttons for frequently called close neighbors, family members and emergency numbers

Here are some ideal questions to ask your loved one:

"Do you need help?"
"What can I do to help you?"
"Do you hurt?"
"Where does it hurt?"

"Are you tired?"
"Do you want to rest?"
"Do you want to sit down?"
"Do you want to lie down?"
"Are you sad?"
"Did someone hurt your feelings?"
"I love you. How can I help you?"

Positive Affirmations

"Love seeks one thing only: the good of the one loved. It leaves all the other secondary effects to take care of themselves. Love, therefore, is its own reward."

– Thomas Merton, Trappist Monk

"Caregivers attract caregivers and live in a community of love. They are energized by their caring, (are) fulfilled, and they love life."

– Gary Zukav, Author

CHAPTER 8

Cognitive (but less complex) Early Warning Signs

"Challenges are what makes life interesting and overcoming them is what makes life meaningful."
– Joshua J. Marine

Laura's Challenges

Laura's cognitive symptoms early in the mild stage were very subtle. Casual friends and acquaintances almost always had no perception that anything was wrong. Close friends and family usually did not recognize anything was amiss or simply attributed any changes in Laura's cognition to getting older. She very effectively used her intelligence to compensate for deficiencies.

By the end of the mild stage, however, Laura began performing poorly in her home life and social environment. She eventually became unable to perform tasks that used to be routine. She was unable to add or subtract figures correctly where previously she could easily do most calculations in her head. Formerly, Laura could remember dozens of telephone numbers, but now she had to ask me to look up and dial the numbers. She had difficulty organizing the times and dates of our appointments, following recipes, balancing our checkbook, handling money and managing routine affairs.

The cognitive but less complex type symptoms usually start off as simply being more forgetful, feeling confused at times and being uneasy. They also include mild memory loss such as difficulty recalling recent events. Learning new information is included with the less complex type symptoms because the first part of the brain that is affected is often memory and learning. Laura also forgot people's names or where she had put things.

Recent Memory Loss

The loved one begins to experience memory loss and starts to have difficulty in remembering recent events. Both short term and new memories are forgotten most quickly. The memory issues involve both recent memory storage and recent memory retrieval. However, pockets of older memories are still present and these are often triggered by familiar faces, voices, smells, touches, music, songs or rituals.

Here are some recent memory loss symptom descriptions:

- Losing, misplacing, and forgetting things gradually becomes common
- Looking for something that you placed somewhere but can't find it
- Sometimes being easily distracted
- Forgetting where you parked the car occurs with more frequency
- Having problems recalling things that happened recently
- From time to time, becoming more forgetful of details of recent events
- Sometimes misplacing items that are commonly used every day
- At times, learning that reading glasses, keys or wallet are not in their usual locations at home
- From time to time, losing or misplacing valuable possessions
- Sporadically believing that someone is intentionally hiding personal items

- Blaming others for stealing lost items
- In some cases, hiding valuables in safe places and then for-getting where they are
- At times, placing things in odd, unusual or strange places like placing keys in the freezer
- Every now and then, placing pantry items in the refrigerator and placing refrigerator items in the pantry
- Sometimes learning that personal toiletry items can't be found
- Occasionally paying for an article at the store and leaving the credit card on the counter
- At times, putting your purse, sweater, or jacket on a chair next to your table in the restaurant and leaving without it
- Sometimes having to look for something that was misplaced
- Making and leaving reminder notes but forget writing them
- At times, forgetting to take daily medications
- Intermittently finding that recent information is fuzzy and not clear or distinct

What Worked for Us That May Work for You

- Decide on routine and consistent places to keep everyday bags, wallets, keys and glasses
- Keeping bathroom items in a small basket or caddy on top of the vanity in plain sight
- Use seven-day medication pill organizers for daily morning and evening medications

Orientation to Time

The loved one starts to become disoriented with the concept of time. For instance, following a hospital stay, loved ones living with dementia are often confused about the time. Here are some time disorientation symptom descriptions:

- Beginning to have trouble or difficulty setting, managing and meeting appointment times
- Occasionally showing confusion about activities involving time and sometimes being disoriented about many aspects of time
- At times, having trouble or difficulty remembering the time to leave for personal care appointments, routine doctor appointments, and entertainment events
- Sporadically needing to be reminded to complete necessary shopping during store operating hours
- Losing track of the current time, the day of the week, today's date and what month, season and year it is
- Sometimes being confused about activities involving time

What Worked for Us That May Work for You

- Obtain a large clock with large numerals and display it prominently
- Obtain a large calendar, note all appointments and other important dates and display it prominently
- Consider placing a white board and mark it up with daily appointments, chores or goals

Orientation to Place

Your loved one may start to become disoriented with the concept of place. Following a hospital stay, the loved one living with dementia often becomes disoriented and can become lost, even in a familiar environment. Here are some place disorientation symptom descriptions:

- Occasionally being confused about location, getting lost or not knowing where you are even in a familiar place
- Sometimes being disoriented and having trouble retaining a sense of direction even in a once familiar neighborhood or place

- Occasionally being disoriented and having trouble retaining a sense of direction in an unfamiliar neighborhood or place
- At times, getting lost going to and returning from familiar locations such as the store
- In some cases, getting lost going to and returning from unfamiliar locations
- Sporadically having difficulty retracing steps
- Having difficulty locating a vehicle in a large parking lot. This can happen especially when mall shopping after entering a store with multiple entrances and then using a different exit. This increases the difficulty locating the parked vehicle

What Worked for Us That May Work for You

- Get in the habit of parking in the same location when shopping at frequently visited stores, such as the supermarket or a mall
- Hold your loved one's hand while walking
- Obtain GPS devices for wrists, ankles, wallets and shoes
- Consider enrolling your loved one in your local community's initiatives to locate special needs individuals when they are lost or disappear

Planning, Organizing and Completing Familiar or Routine Tasks

The loved one starts to have difficulty performing familiar or everyday tasks or chores that were once easily performed. The procedural memory becomes degraded and the ability to remember and retrieve processes is more difficult. Here is some dysfunctional planning, organizing and completing tasks symptom descriptions:

- Sometimes managing everyday technology becomes difficult
- Occasionally having trouble following simple recipes and cooking a meal

- At times, being confused by even simple things in your home including microwave oven, stovetop, oven, dishwasher, washer, dryer, vacuum cleaner, steam iron, television remote control, security alarm, telephone answering machine or device, and the alarm clock
- Sometimes forgetting to flush the toilet or turn off the faucet
- Your loved one's personal appearance sometimes ranges from very neat to barely presentable

What Worked for Us That May Work for You

- Convert your home computer to the simplest notebook type and offer your loved one continual help on how to use it
- Cheerfully take over the operation and use of all appliances

Declining Judgment and Poor Judgment:
Here are some "poor judgment" symptom descriptions:

- Sometimes making poor decisions concerning financial matters
- Sporadically helping or enabling family members or friends who normally should be treated with tough love
- At times, having trouble or difficulty making decisions and prefer to defer to others
- Occasionally permitting door-to-door sales people to enter your home
- From time to time, authorizing unlicensed repair people who were previously unknown to you – and not recommended by friends or family members – to perform work on your home
- Sometimes signing up for new but unwanted magazine subscriptions and renewing existing subscriptions for many years in the future
- Occasionally talking to telemarketers on the phone and being influenced by their sales pitch

- At times, ordering unneeded, unnecessary or excessive items from television sales pitches
- Sometimes making major decisions that impact your future life and are suspect to your loved ones
- Wanting to change your marital status for no reason
- Sometimes communicating unrealistic judgments or unrealistic expectations

What Worked for Us That May Work for You

- Offer help, consultation, discussion of alternatives and assistance as a team member
- Research and take the steps to eliminate junk mail offers and catalogs
- Convert your home telephone to a type that can block telemarketer calls
- Place a no solicitation sign on the front door

Focus, Attention and Concentration

Here are some dysfunctional focus, attention and concentration symptom descriptions:

- Occasionally, when retrieving something, walking into a different room and then realizing that you can't remember why or what is the purpose of the search
- In some cases, having brain fog and senior moments when thinking
- Sometimes becoming easily distracted
- At times, forgetting where you parked the car
- Occasionally opening the door to the pantry or refrigerator at home then forgetting what item is being sought
- Having difficulty being flexible and readily accepting changes
- In some cases, adapting and thriving becomes difficult
- At times, having difficulty recognizing familiar faces or objects

- Being more and more confused for no reason.
- Every so often, having trouble or difficulty remembering the name of a person who has just been introduced
- Sometimes having trouble or difficulty remembering the name of a store just visited
- Having trouble or difficulty remembering to take personal medications unless reminded
- Needing to be reminded to accomplish normal household chores or tasks
- Trouble or difficulty remembering important dates like birthdays, anniversaries or family gatherings
- Being more forgetful is becoming common
- Sporadically becoming absent minded
- Sometimes having decreased concentration
- Occasionally having difficulty focusing attention
- Sometimes having a greatly decreased attention span; not reading books, not watching movies or insisting to leave a play at intermission

What Worked for Us That May Work for You

- Accept your loved one's deficiencies and strive to minimize these issues
- Patience and understanding become more important caregiver requirements as the disease progressives

Positive Affirmations

"Gratitude helps us to see what is there instead of what isn't."
– *Annette Bridges*

"A positive attitude may not solve all your problems, but it will annoy enough people to make it worth the effort." – *Herm Albright*

"The beginning of anxiety is the end of faith, and the beginning of true faith is the end of anxiety." – *George E. Mueller*

"To care for those who once cared for us is one of the highest honors." – *Tia Walker*

CHAPTER 9

Cognitive (but more complex) Early Warning Signs

"And once the storm is over, you won't remember how you made it through, how you managed to survive. You won't even be sure whether the storm is over. But one thing is certain. When you come out of the storm, you won't be the same person who walked in. That's what this storm's all about."
– Haruki Murakami

When we downsized from a home with over 3,300 square feet to one that had 2,200 square feet, we moved the small items ourselves and used a professional mover for the large and heavy items. This was our tenth residence since we were married, so Laura was well familiar with moving and organizing a kitchen.

Laura's Challenges

But Laura was at a loss on how to do this one.

Naturally, I lined all the cabinets as this was always a priority for Laura. But where to put what? I really had no idea, so, we asked our daughter to help and she had the job done in no time. I was too busy with other details of moving to think about the implications of this event. But I did realize it was totally unlike Laura to let some other woman (even our daughter) make decisions about the kitchen set-up. The kitchen was always her domain.

About that time, Laura's pension fund was taken over by a new company for the fourth time since she retired. This time, Laura was given the option to continue her pension or to accept a lump sum payment to spend or roll over to her Individual Retirement Account (IRA). I thought that it didn't matter, so I insisted Laura make the decision. Nope, she deferred that decision to me. Again, this was totally unlike her as she loved being hands-on with her IRA stock choices. Over the years, her decisions were always sound so I supported whatever she decided. But not this time; Laura refused to make the decision. I was baffled at the time and decided not to decide. So, Laura's pension payments were continued as is.

Our new home was formerly the model for the development. As a model, the furnishings looked fantastic. Laura was determined to end up with an equally attractive or more attractive home than the model's décor. So, we employed decorator number one who was soon replaced by decorator number two. Those two ladies were frustrated as they could not finalize their recommendations into a finished product. Finally, we employed decorator number three, who seemed to understand our needs and also had empathy for Laura's current indecisiveness. Her decorator knowledge and social skills were extremely strong so we ended up with a beautifully decorated home at a reasonable cost. I wondered at length about this process as Laura had always taken pride and finalized a beautiful home décor in our previous nine residences without the help of a decorator.

With hindsight, I later realized that Laura could no longer deal with the more complex aspects of planning, organizing and implementing changes involving our new home.

Deterioration of Basic Executive Skills
Laura began to experience deterioration of her basic executive skills, including planning, organizing, delegating, initiating, following-up and completing tasks.

Here are some planning/organizing symptom descriptions:

- Sometimes becoming distracted and tending to avoid problematic issues
- Occasionally having difficulty or trouble completing familiar or routine tasks at home or work and in social or leisure activities
- At times, getting frustrated and quitting tasks that were once easily accomplished
- Randomly having difficulty or trouble carrying out simple instructions
- From time to time, withdrawing from mental challenges when it has become difficult to accomplish logical thinking
- At times, procrastinating becomes somewhat common
- Having difficulty handling money
- Struggling with familiar daily tasks such as managing finances like the household budget, pension and bank accounts
- Occasionally having difficulty planning grocery shopping
- Randomly having trouble or difficulty following recipes to prepare the main course or side courses of a meal
- From time to time, having trouble or difficulty organizing a family gathering
- Every so often, having trouble or difficulty setting the dining room table for a family meal
- At times, having trouble or difficulty following a lengthy or complex recipe
- Occasionally forgetting to turn off the burner on the stove
- Occasionally, starting to have difficulty in the sequence or order of putting on clothes.
- At times, having trouble or difficulty refilling prescriptions, taking daily medications, and tracking medications already taken
- Changing the current time on clocks when daylight saving time changes is difficult

- Forgetting to keep doors and windows locked and the security alarm on
- Sometimes, losing initiative to start various projects at home or work
- Occasionally, finding it difficult to start a project in your yard although you enjoy being outside to cut the grass or work in your flower beds

What Worked for Us That May Work for You

- Remove the burner knobs from the stove when necessary
- Unplug the electrical 220V cord for the electric stove receptacle
- Partnering and assisting the loved one on once familiar chores becomes commonplace. It is vital to permit the loved one to handle as many tasks as they are able to if they can. The sense of accomplishment and personal pride from completing small tasks is fulfilling for the loved one.

Deterioration of More Advanced Executive Skills

Laura started to experience deterioration of the more advanced executive skills of planning, organizing, delegating, initiating, following-up and completing a new or more complex task. She could no longer stay focused on it. Here are some new/complex task planning, organizing symptom descriptions:

- Sometimes, having difficulty or trouble making future plans, setting goals and organizing future events
- Making then changing or cancelling long-term plans because of difficulty comprehending the mechanics of execution
- At times, having difficulty or trouble delegating assignments to others and initiating the start of the activity as well as following-up on the activity and solving problems as they become apparent

- Every so often, having difficulty learning from consequences of past actions and modifying future actions
- At times, having difficulty multi-tasking when involved in more complex projects
- Occasionally becoming easily distracted and intentionally avoiding problematic issues
- Having trouble or difficulty understanding instructions containing a sequence of steps
- Sometimes, having trouble or difficulty gathering the detailed information necessary to complete and actually completing the annual tax return
- Sometimes, being slower to grasp new or complex ideas
- Occasionally, having difficulty concentrating and thinking things through
- Decreased motivation and initiative to start various projects at home or work
- At times, procrastinating and avoiding being involved in changes planned by another
- From time to time, being less productive at work because of its complex, challenging and difficult requirements

What Worked for Us That May Work for You

- Employ teamwork to assist the loved one in completing daily chores, make short-term plans and enjoy local activities
- Communicate with your loved one in an understanding and patient way, realizing that the processing speed for a person living with dementia slows considerably

Judgment and Decision-Making Functions

Laura began to experience declines in the areas of common-sense judgment and logical decision making. Here are some judgment/decision making symptom descriptions:

- Occasionally relying on others to make decisions that used to be easily handled alone
- At times, uncertainty and hesitancy begins to occur
- Procrastinating on initiating action
- Sometimes having to rely on someone else to keep up with appointments and events
- Having reduced use of reason, logic and judgment
- Sporadically using creative fibbing during doctor visits and convincing the primary medical provider that nothing is wrong
- Refusing to see a specialist after the primary doctor makes a referral. The rationale and excuses used are: "They only want our money! There is nothing wrong with me."

What Worked for Us That May Work for You

- Have the Power of Attorney for Financial Matters completed and/or updated on a high priority basis?
- Place a credit freeze at all three credit bureaus for the loved one living with dementia
- Never disclose to a caller that a person living with dementia lives in your home and could possibly answer the telephone. This would result in a possible scam caller obtaining that fact and then selling your telephone number to other scam ventures
- Set up caller ID on home and cell phones to only accept calls from callers that transmit their name and telephone number. Screen calls and ignore all calls without a name or telephone number provided
- Do not answer calls from area codes that are unfamiliar or you do not recognize
- Use an iPad or computer to perform an internet search on unusual area codes and unusual ten-digit numbers. Many times, you will easily determine that it is a scam number or a number that has had hundreds of searches previously by others

- Disconnect your answering machine or answering/recording capabilities. Let calls simply ring and ring during the day when you are away from the phone. Eventually, the computer robot machine will drop your number
- The person living with dementia becomes a prime candidate for scam artists. Modern times, modern crimes. Once the crooks determine a person with dementia lives in the home, they will attack continually by telephone, email, US mail, or even personal front-door solicitations

Arithmetical Reasoning and Problem Solving

Laura began to have difficulty performing calculations, handling money and managing financial affairs. Her ability to remember meanings and use her acquired mathematical knowledge was slowly lost. Here are some arithmetical reasoning symptom descriptions:

- Sporadically having trouble or difficulty managing money, calculating tips or calculating the correct change to be returned by the cashier
- Having trouble or difficulty paying the monthly bills on time
- Randomly, having trouble or difficulty remembering how to manage finances and investments
- Finding it difficult to perform simple arithmetic problems
- At times, finding it difficult to perform simple pencil and paper arithmetic in your head and without using a calculator
- Having trouble balancing the household budget such as income and expenses
- Occasionally writing checks that exceed the balance available
- At time, having trouble remembering personal home or cell phone numbers, social security numbers and dates of birth of self, spouse or children
- Sometimes accepting the bank statement as always accurate because, "The bank never makes mistakes"

What Worked for Us That May Work for You

- Gradually take over the financial affairs of your loved one
- Keep hard copy files of important financial information

Learning New Information

Laura had difficulty learning new, revised and additional information. Here are some learning new information symptom descriptions:

- Sometimes grasping new ideas or solving problems is difficult
- At times, managing everyday technology has become difficult
- Difficulty interpreting, learning and retaining new and unfamiliar information
- Occasionally having trouble or difficulty concentrating and learning new things or how to use new electronic gadgets

What Worked for Us That May Work for You

- Avoid introducing new technology to your loved one. Try to continue using whatever technology is in your loved one's comfort zone

Perceptual Abilities Become Degraded

The loved one has more difficulty perceiving the world around them as it really exists. Here are some perceptual abilities symptom descriptions:

- Sometimes the television becomes a window to the world in that your loved one believes what is happening on the screen is happening just outside your home
- Occasionally, when a fire truck, police car or ambulance siren is heard, it is perceived as coming to your home

What Worked for Us That May Work for You

- Keep the television and the radio off when both become problematic and upset your loved one

Abstraction Thinking Abilities Become Degraded

Laura started to have problems with abstract thinking. The ability to make the leap from symbolic thinking to the real world was slowly lost. Here are some abstract thinking symptom descriptions:

- Randomly having problems with abstract thinking and discussions
- Occasionally beginning to have difficulty understanding abstract concepts like bravery, kindness, empathy, courage, or cowardice
- Difficulty thinking about and discussing emotions like love, hate, happiness, or sadness. Concepts like justice, peace and freedom are lost
- Randomly not clearly understanding metaphors to describe an angry person like "He is a raging bull"
- At times, not clearly understanding similes like "as boring as watching paint dry"
- Not understanding analogies like "pretty as a picture" to describe an attractive person
- Sometimes finding difficultly discussing alternative vacation plans for next summer
- Learning that it is difficult discussing and understanding how children are educated in foreign countries is relevant to the education of children in our country
- Finding it is difficult discussing and understanding the alternatives that will have to be faced when a spouse dies

What Worked for Us That May Work for You

- Keeping the loved one living with dementia socially engaged
- Helping he or she use their brain for problem solving
- Continuing to enjoy regular daily activities
- Live each day to the fullest
- Kindness and gratitude motivate positive thoughts and will lift you up
- Appreciate life even more after becoming a caregiver

Positive Affirmations

"Most of the important things in the world have been accomplished by people who kept on trying when there seemed to be no hope at all." – *Dale Carnegie*

"The simple act of caring is heroic." – *Edward Albert, actor*

"Caring for our seniors is perhaps the greatest responsibility we have. Those who walked before us have given so much and made possible the life we all enjoy." – *Senator John Hoeven*

CHAPTER 10

Physical Early Warning Signs

"Offering care means being a companion, not a superior. It doesn't matter whether the person we are caring for is experiencing cancer, the flu, dementia, or grief. If you are a doctor or surgeon, your expertise and knowledge come from a superior position. But when our role is to be providers of care, we should be there as equals."
– Judy Cornish

Visual Spatial Issues

Like most people, Laura has had a lifetime fear of falling from high places. Imagine Laura or yourself in this situation:

Let's say we are both on a roof top of a twenty-story building, and I ask Laura to stand at the edge of the roof with her toes over the edge. Since Laura trusts me, she does it. Laura is now standing with her toes slightly over the edge, looking down to the ground far below. She has a queasy feeling about being so high in this potentially life-threatening situation. Laura then starts to imagine falling twenty stories! "Don't look down!" I forcefully instruct. But she does. It gives her a sick feeling looking down when she was so high up. Everything on the ground looks tiny to Laura. She has always feared heights. Laura feels more fear than she has ever felt in her life. Her survival instinct tells her not to step forward, not to fall from this high building. It tells her to freeze and then slowly and carefully back up away from the dangerous edge of this building. Desperately, Laura tries to back away from the edge but cannot as someone behind her is exerting slight pressure on her back. The person behind her is clearly irritated and is assertively speaking words that may be in a foreign language. But Laura doesn't understand a word that person behind her is saying. She then hears me say in clear English, "Take one step forward. You must do it now! We are in a hurry! Please step forward and down one step!" Laura has full trust in me and my voice has a sense of urgency. But Laura's fright turns into terror. She screams, "NO! I WON'T DO IT! NO!"

Now you know how Laura felt just before she exited the passenger car of a train in Europe.

After we both retired, Laura and I started traveling to Europe. We loved to travel, see unfamiliar places, explore new cities, meet new people and experience new cultures. Each self-guided trip was a unique and treasured adventure. After studying the benefits of Eurail passes and promising Laura that all would go well, I purchased a three-country Eurail travel package to visit France, Germany and Austria. Traveling by rail between large European cities is highly preferable to rental car travel. We knew we would enjoy this adventure and have a similar itinerary that professional travel tours offer but at half the cost. The savings meant we could do twice the travel for the same money. Laura and I also enjoyed the adventure of being on our own in a foreign country even though we only knew a few words of the language. Laura has never met a stranger and always finds things to talk about with the people she meets, so finding Europeans who wish to chat and practice their English was never a problem. Little did I know about the real adventure we would have on this trip.

This was the first time I became aware of Laura's visual/spatial issues. This condition is called visual spatial perceptual difficulties. In the beginning, it was severe depth perception difficulties. It is clearly a challenging behavior for Laura and is often the earliest sign of physical issues caused by dementia. However, at the time I was unaware of that possibility and thought it was simply a new vision problem.

Here's what happened. We were beginning our rail trip after flying to Germany and accessed the train without an issue. Naturally, there are train connections/transfers to make and train schedules to meet. At our first train connection/transfer, I exited the passenger car at the station. Struggling with our luggage, I offloaded one large suitcase at a time then turned around and asked Laura to come next. There were only three descending steps to take. She froze as if her feet were glued to the floor. She started breathing heavily. Her face blanched. She shouted, "NO! I WON'T DO IT! NO!" It was clear to me that she was having something like a panic attack.

The European trains run on time and we had to change from this train to another at this station. The people behind Laura were obviously becoming irritated as they also might miss their train transfer. I shifted from urgency to calmness in my speech, telling Laura that we were just exiting the train and there were grab rails on each side of the steps. I kept repeating that I knew she could do it. I kept my voice low, relaxed, calm and controlled. She remained frozen at the top of the passenger car exit. I asked for her hand bag and day bag and offloaded both of them near our suitcases. This freed up both of Laura's hands. I put her hands on the grab rails and she tightly gripped them. I touched her right foot and said that she must move this foot one step lower. I calmly repeated it several times. I then placed my hands under her armpits and supported her as she accomplished this first step and she got her right foot down. I gave her warm praise as feedback. Then I asked her to move the other foot down to that step. We repeated this process until we got off the train. "Whew!" I thought. "This trip will be an adventure!" The trip lasted for two weeks and included three major all-day rides, each with at least one transfer. We also visited the Czech Republic on separate train rides not included in the Eurail package.

I learned how to calm Laura to overcome her fear of using steps to exit the passenger cars. We were eventually successful, as passengers behind us usually recognized the problem, were sympathetic and assisted or called the train conductor to assist.

On that trip, the issue included a new difficulty: Descending steps to access subway/metro/commuter train platforms. Laura would tightly grip the stairway handrail and slowly and carefully descend the steps. Since we had the appearance of being feeble and handicapped, we became magnets for the hordes of petty criminals and pickpockets that ply their trade in crowded tourist areas. But we were seasoned travelers, so our valuables were always safe under our clothes hanging from secure bags around our necks. However, I was aware of the petty thieves and experienced my buttocks being felt up in my rear wallet pocket area several times.

Western Europe is not as handicapped-friendly as the U.S., so I learned where elevators were located in all the multi-story buildings where we shopped, the buildings that we visited as tourist attractions and in train terminals.

Laura continued this fear even after we returned home. She would carefully descend from our home's upper level, taking one step at a time while tightly gripping the stairway bannister.

Thinking the issue could have been caused by bifocal eyeglasses, Laura's eyes were examined and new progressive lens glasses were prescribed and purchased. That didn't help, so we next tried cataract surgery on both her eyes. That didn't help either. Then new eyeglasses again. That also didn't help, but the eyewear provider loved us because Laura only selected stylish, expensive and prestigious name-brand frames. Laura's shopping instincts for quality goods were as sharp as ever.

Laura's issue soon included avoiding all downward escalators. She absolutely would not enter a downward escalator. Later, the difficulty extended to upward escalators. Yet, we did not stop traveling. Instead, we adjusted. I learned the location of every elevator in our home city and in every multi-story building we visited while traveling stateside and to Europe for the next decade.

Did I suspect that Laura had mild dementia? No, absolutely not.

I simply thought it was some unique vision or balance problem associated with aging that we both had to accept. How did our optometrist miss the fact that Laura had mild dementia? How did our primary medical provider that does our six-month check-ups miss Laura's mild dementia? How did the specialist who investigated her balance problems miss it also? At the time, I remained in the dark and did the best I could.

We traveled for many years during Laura's mild dementia progression. But life goes on after dementia strikes. It's just different. Laura enjoyed traveling and so did I. In hindsight, I now know that this trip marked Laura's entrance into mild dementia.

Some Background Information

As a caregiver, you must understand what your loved one sees and how it relates to their spatial relationship. Both the images seen and the perception of the size and location of surroundings are real to your loved one. In doctor's offices, standard tests to measure the degree of dementia include several drawings to evaluate the decline of visual/spatial abilities. Some of the simple figure drawing are three dimensional and some are two dimensional. They work to establish a baseline in order to follow the visual/spatial decline as it progresses.

Visual/spatial difficulties are extremely difficult for caregivers to clearly comprehend. Caregivers must simply do the best they can knowing that it will never be good enough. Help, support and reassurance will help your loved one feel safe.

As a caregiver, you will need to understand that your loved one is seeing things less sharply, distorted and in a blurry format. Often, their vision is shadowed from small shapes floating in the visual field. Loss of peripheral vision or side to side vision is common as the visual field becomes smaller. Judging distances to an object and seeing that object in three dimensions greatly deteriorates.

Color perception will be impacted. The elementary school memory aid, ROY G BIV is an abbreviation for the color spectrum red, orange, yellow, green, blue, indigo and violet. The vision of the loved one living with dementia will be best on the red to green spectrum. Conversely, the loved one will have great difficulty seeing the blue to violet spectrum. For example, he or she will easily see red strawberries, yellow squash and green broccoli on a red plate. However, blueberries and blackberries on a dark blue plate will be nearly invisible. Seeing white mashed potatoes on a white plate may be impossible.

Here are some ideas to consider when it comes to color or light misperception ...

- Consider using a red toilet seat to make it easier to see
- Consider using red plates on a white tablecloth. It is much easier for the loved one to see than a white plate on a white tablecloth
- Try to avoid busy patterns and changes in floor patterns or surfaces. They may be seen as an obstacle or barrier and may be avoided
- Your loved one may need more time to adapt to changes in light levels such as when going from a bright room to a dark room. Naturally, bedroom and bathroom night lights should be in the red, orange, or yellow spectrum and not in the blue, indigo or violet shades
- The loved one may have problems positioning themselves on a chair or on the toilet. The room may be too bright to navigate or too busy and confusing due to patterned wallpaper.

If your loved one living with dementia lives at home, it may not be clear how their visual difficulties affect them until they experience a change in environment. This could include visiting family, going shopping or going on vacation.

Continue routine eye care. Schedule regular eye check-ups and privately inform the optometrist and assistant of the loved one's dementia. A skilled optometrist can complete a comprehensive exam without the use of alphabetical eye charts. How? They use other charts of simple drawings. For example, a simple drawing of a birthday cake is often used. They understand that the loved one's processing speed is much slower so they compensate by taking additional time for the examination.

Make certain that the loved one wears the correct glasses for a specific activity, such as reading. Either label the glasses or have a different color frame for different activities like red frames for reading and black frames for watching television.

Multifocal glasses can increase the risk of falls when loved ones are outside the home. It may be beneficial to have separate glasses for distance (usually worn outside) and for reading (in the home). Many people take off multifocal glasses when ascending or descending steps.

If your loved one fails to recognize an object, don't draw any unnecessary attention to the mistake. Avoid asking questions that might make them feel put on the spot. If appropriate, give the object to the person and explain how it is used. If they do not accept this explanation, try not to argue with them. Ignore the mistake and listen to what they are trying to say. Being corrected can undermine a loved one's confidence, and he or she may become reluctant to join in conversations or activities. Therefore, it is important to focus on the emotions behind what is being said, rather than the facts or details.

Recognizing the Physical Symptoms

Early physical signs of dementia may be mild, but they may be recognized as they occur frequently and sometimes repeatedly, constantly and consistently. These minor problems can happen seldom or often, even every waking hour of every day.

The early warning signs of physical symptoms come in many different forms and, while some of them are easily recognizable, others can slip by unnoticed. Unfortunately, there is no absolute set or concrete pattern of symptoms to inform a lay person exactly how far along a loved one living with dementia is or what specific form of dementia they are experiencing.

As soon as you notice mild early warning signs of the physical symptoms of dementia, contact your doctor for a checkup. The sooner the disease is recognized, the earlier the caregiver may begin planning for the future. Symptoms usually start off small such as being more forgetful, repeating things, trouble sleeping, feeling confused and being uneasy.

Laura's Challenges

Dealing with the physical symptoms is somewhat challenging but can be properly handled with the correct direct interaction. Here are some early warning signs involving physical symptoms of dementia which could leave to a higher potential for falling:

- Occasionally having more physical weakness and difficulty opening twist off lids or caps
- Sometimes walking slower with a shorter step or gait
- Sporadically having muscle twitching, especially in bed during sleep
- Constantly having visual/spatial difficulty using downward stairs
- At times, having difficulty recognizing and understanding visual images and related spatial relationships
- Experiencing deterioration of three-dimensional and peripheral vision
- Sometimes having diminished ability to smell unpleasant and pleasant odors
- Difficulty in hearing and understanding a nearby person in a large, noisy room
- Occasionally misinterpreting patterns or reflections in mirrors
- Sometimes napping more during the day and being awake at night
- Sometimes engaging in repetitive physical activity
- Having less ability to taste food as taste buds change, such as becoming more or less sensitive to sweet and sour tastes

What Worked for Us That May Work for You

- The increased togetherness was a good thing for both of us. Dementia actually rejuvenated our marriage. We were never the couple who goes out to eat, sits at the restaurant table and doesn't speak to one another or who stare at their cell phones during the entire dinner
- I kept Laura socially engaged, helping her use her brain for problem solving
- I initiated many, diverse, walking adventures. We walked in our home, danced in our home, walked in our neighborhood and in parks. We took extra shopping trips. We went to many local college activities and were regulars at our community's stage shows. Laura and my individual retirement activities diminished, but our activities together greatly increased. The volunteers at local activities and stage show were always willing to help me get Laura up and down steps
- We increased our socialization with family, friends and neighbors. We gave parties and went to parties. We attended community meetings and were regulars in church activities
- We sought out group activities and classes. Dancing lessons were our favorite
- I made it a priority to reduce Laura's risk of falling
- I began to make the home environment safer
- I equipped stairs and steps with double railings or bannisters
- I equipped bathtubs, showers and toilets with grab rails
- I equipped entrance and exit doors with grab bars
- I eliminated loose throw rugs
- I gradually simplified the home and reduced the number of items on countertops
- I removed the shower doors and converted the showers to a walk-in for ease of access and egress
- I included a shower bench and converted the shower nozzle to a handheld wand

- Laura and I walked for exercise which generated many physical and emotional health benefits
- We purchased small quantities of groceries each day and walked the perimeter of the store
- We window shopped when mall walking in inclement weather

Positive Affirmations

"Physical activity is an excellent stress-buster and provides other health benefits as well. It can improve your mood and self-image." – *Jon Wickham*

"My caregiver mantra is to remember: The only control you have is over the changes you choose to make." – *Nancy L. Kriseman*

"To enjoy the glow of good health, you must exercise." – *Gene Tunney*

"Increased physical activity enhances positive energy." – *Lailah Gifty Akita*

"Gratitude helps us to see what is there instead of what isn't." – *Annette Bridges*

"The reason I exercise is for the quality of life I enjoy." – *Kenneth H. Cooper*

"Fitness is not about being better than someone else...It's about being better than you used to be." – *Khloe Kardashian*

"Strength does not come from physical capacity. It comes from an indomitable will." – *Mahatma Gandhi*

CHAPTER 11

Emotional Early Warning Signs

"Better a diamond with a flaw than a pebble without one."
– Chinese Proverb

Laura experienced social anxiety when she entered mild dementia. This was difficult for me to understand because her normal personality was outgoing and highly social. Early in our retirement years, we played bridge at every opportunity. It was a wonderful way to meet nice people in our age range and social group. But after the dementia began, Laura became more and more reluctant to engage in bridge games. Eventually, she would only partner with me because she was not comfortable getting constructive and/or negative feedback when we rotated partnering with others. I did not understand her viewpoint but accepted it to keep Laura happy.

Laura sometimes became offended by relatives, friends and neighbors when given any form of negative or constructive feedback. The give and take aspects of normal conversation seemed to have become too complex. She would then avoid contact with that person or any situation where that person was present.

At the time, I did not understand why Laura was bothered by these issues. They seemed minor to me so I tried to smooth them over to the best of my ability. With hindsight, I now understand that

Laura had entered the mild stage of dementia and these were simply emotional early warning signs of the disease.

Recognizing the Symptoms

Emotional and personality symptoms are also called the Behavioral and Psychological Symptoms of Dementia (BPSD). These challenges or symptoms are the feelings and emotions that the loved one living with dementia experiences. A more technical term is the affective challenges. Another specialized term is dysphoria, which is a state of generalized unhappiness, restlessness, dissatisfaction or frustration.

It is important that the state of dysphoria, the affective challenges and the BPSD terms be understood. These technical terms are common in the language of the medical community. Caregivers should be familiar with these terms to better communicate with the primary care physician and with specialists when referrals are necessary.

In my experience, it is not important for the caregiver to differentiate between behavioral symptoms and psychological symptoms. Nor is it important to have a detailed knowledge of each symptom.

It is important, however, to realize that no two people with dementia have an identical progression of the disease. Also, in the early or mild stage, people with different dementia diseases have widely different emotional symptoms and behaviors. In the mild stage, the challenges of the emotional symptoms are the least difficult to manage. For the typical person living with dementia, these challenges are common and somewhat upsetting but easily manageable.

Very few people in the early stages are diagnosed with dementia because of the mildness of the emotional symptoms. The symptoms are usually accepted as a normal consequence of aging. Essentially, a normal life continues for the caregiver and the loved one living with dementia. This was true for Laura and me. We simply ignored the symptoms, continued our rewarding life and tried our best to enjoy our retirement years.

As soon as you notice that the mild behavioral changes in personality are becoming difficult for your loved one or yourself, contact your doctor for a checkup. The sooner the disease is recognized, the earlier the caregiver may begin planning for the future.

The following general behavior symptoms that impacted Laura are listed to help you better understand the emotional warning signs of dementia. I list these using hindsight, as at the time I did not understand them.

Laura's Challenges

Mood, personality and emotional changes:

- At times, Laura had rapid mood swings
- Sometimes she showed more emotion than previously for a relatively minor matter
- Occasionally, she had more difficulty controlling emotions such as fear, sadness, anger and irritability
- Often had a reduced sense of humor
- Sporadically became more stubborn or rigid
- Sometimes uncharacteristically insistent on having her way
- At times, Laura was unwilling to consider the views of others

Deterioration of social graces, norms, tact and empathy to others:

- Her social skills reduced and she began social withdrawal
- Sometimes close family and friends complained that Laura was no longer the same person
- She became easily offended by others when no offense was intended
- Often no longer had quick come-backs to social slights from others
- She no longer used humor to defuse stressful situations

- Laura was less concerned about how her words affected others
- Sometimes became offended by a close loved one over something minor and remained offended for an unusually long time
- Had negative thoughts about a loved one and expressed them to others

Becoming suspicious and experiencing paranoia:

- Sometimes had trouble finding car keys or reading glasses and blamed others
- Every now and then, Laura hid her wallet, pocketbook, checkbook and other personal items in a location at home and then had difficulty finding them
- At times, believed that someone was intentionally hiding or stealing her personal items
- Sometimes was suspicious about the intentions or motives of other people

Experiencing marital suspicions:

- Sometimes, Laura subtly questioned me about members of the opposite sex and the accusation of possible perceived infidelity was clear
- Occasionally had a false belief that I was insincere, possibly disloyal and was no longer deeply in love with her
- Sporadically thought and voiced suspicions that I was interested in greener pastures

Having unusual repetitive activity:

- At times, excessive and unnecessary physical activity began although the symptoms were minor like opening and closing drawers repeatedly

- Sometimes Laura walked into a room to search for an item but forgot the reason
- She abandoned the search but later repeated the activity with the same result
- From time to time, she opened and closed her pocketbook or wallet as if looking for something but never found it

Having agitation:

- Sometimes Laura became verbally confrontational, lost composure and became upset over minor issues
- At times, she became angry and frustrated because she had trouble doing the what she used to do
- Sporadically lashed out to family members due to small problems
- Laura felt agitated and no longer in control of simple daily tasks and activities
- Occasionally was anxious, irritable, stubborn, agitated or temperamental
- At times, she was unreasonably or uncharacteristically argumentative

Having some depression:

- Sometimes changed from having a positive, upbeat and happy attitude to being negative, downcast and sad
- Occasionally became tearful without a seemingly good reason
- Experienced pleasurable activities less and couldn't relax
- At times, was anxious or worried about events that are routine

Experiencing apathy and lack of initiative:

- At times, intentionally avoided people and withdrew from social challenges or events

- Occasionally was more passive and less motivated to try new activities
- Sometimes lacked curiosity about topics that would usually have been highly interesting
- From time to time, was less likely to initiate or maintain conversation
- Laura became less affectionate

What Worked for Us That May Work for You

- I addressed Laura's behavior in a positive manner, using a person-centered approach
- I kept Laura socially engaged and continuing to enjoy regular daily activities
- We tried to live each day to the fullest
- I would smooth over frustrating conversations using humor, distraction, changing the subject and changing the location
- I found that a smile and a cheerful tone provided the body language that facilitated an improved attitude
- After I used something, I left it where it was or in a familiar place. I followed the adage: A place for everything, and everything in its place

Positive Affirmations

"If you can't change your fate, change your attitude."
– *Amy Tan*

"Caring is doing what has to be done and not expecting anything in return." – *thecaregiverspace.org*

CHAPTER 12

Do It Yourself Mild Dementia Diagnosis

"You don't develop courage by being happy in your relationships every day. You develop it by surviving difficult times and challenging adversity."
– Epicurus

Laura's cognitive symptoms early in the mild stage were subtle. The early changes she experienced began gradually with mild memory loss. Laura had difficulty recalling recent events and learning new information. She sometimes forgot people's names and where she may have put things. I did not suspect that she had started on the downward slope of dementia progression. Close friends and family did not recognize anything was amiss. Casual friends and acquaintances had no perception anything was wrong. Laura very effectively used her intelligence to compensate for deficiencies.

However, by the end of the mild stage, Laura begin performing poorly at housework, social life and at home. She eventually became unable to perform tasks that used to be routine in her daily life. She was unable to add or subtract figures correctly, where previously she was skilled. Formerly, Laura could remember dozens of telephone numbers but now she had to ask me to look up and dial the numbers. She had difficulty organizing times and dates, following recipes, balancing our checkbook, handling money and managing routine affairs. I then clearly understood that cognitive issues existed and used the internet to learn more about this subject.

Did we discuss Laura's cognitive issues? Yes and no. Whenever I addressed this possibility, I was always met with resistance. Laura would assertively state, "My business is my business and no one else needs to know my business!" When I interjected that it affected me also, her reply was usually, "Our business is our business and no one else needs to know our business!" Her expectations were clear. We were not to discuss it with anyone else nor each other. Yes, Laura preferred secrecy rather than honesty. And, yes, on this issue, Laura was the boss.

Due to the many diverse types of dementia, the early warning signs may come in a wide spectrum of symptoms. In the mild stage, the symptoms vary depending on the different type of dementia being experienced. There is no absolute set of symptoms to guide the progression from normal aging to dementia. However, there are many early symptoms that can be easily recognized and used as an indicator that a physician should be consulted. The medical community firmly believes that timely treatment will result in the lessening of the severity of the symptoms and thereby improve the quality of life for a person living with dementia.

Ten Warning Signs

The U.S. Alzheimer's Associations publishes the ten warning signs. They are republished in the same or similar formats in most countries where the English language is commonly used. They were listed in detail in Chapter 5 and are summarized as follows:

1. Memory loss that disrupts daily life
2. Challenges in planning or solving problems
3. Difficulty completing familiar tasks
4. Confusion with time or place
5. Trouble understanding visual images and spatial relationships

6. New problems with words in speaking or writing
7. Misplacing things and losing the ability to retrace steps
8. Decreased or poor judgment
9. Withdrawal from work or social activities
10. Changes in mood and personality [1]

The Alzheimer's Association also provides a useful document on line entitled, *Tools for Early Identification, Assessment, and Treatment for People with Alzheimer's Disease and Dementia.*

What's Next?

Is it just senior moments and not dementia? Could it be dementia? Is it possibly dementia? Is it probably dementia? Is it certain to be dementia? It is not rocket science to utilize the world's readily available and easy to understand guidelines that will provide answers to these questions.

The paragraphs that follow are my home-made, non-scientific, personal version. Go back through the signs and symptoms listed in chapters 7 through 11. Make a check mark for each statement which is definitely true for your loved one. There are about 250 statements in all. This personal version of mine is not intended to replace a professional diagnosis. However, you can take your marked-up copy of this book to your next clinician visit to refresh your memory and provide input on this subject.

Let's say you use 20 percent or less as your benchmark to guesstimate that your loved one does NOT have mild dementia nor mild cognitive impairment. If so, and if the number of statements you checked is 50 or less, consider them as senior moments and assume your loved one's cognition is normal. However, there's nothing sacred about 20 percent. Use 10 or 30 percent if you prefer.

Between 20 and 70 percent? That means 50 to 175 symptoms are checked. If so, then you can now guesstimate that your loved one may have Mild Cognitive Impairment (MCI). However, since MCI may also progress to dementia, discuss this with your primary care physician during your next routine visit.

And then you can use 70 percent or more to guesstimate that your loved one possibly has dementia. If so, and if the number of statements checked is 175 or more, then it is time to make an appointment to visit your primary care physician. At that visit, focus the discussion on the possibility that your loved one may be living with dementia. As stated above, there's nothing sacred about this percentile as an indication of dementia.

Self-administered tests

Please note that most of these self-administered, brief, online, cognitive tests, questionnaires and forms are protected by copyright. Naturally, that prevents me from including them in this book. However, they are easily accessed on the internet for individual use, so feel free to use them.

Memory Impairment Screen: The MIS is a brief screening tool to assess short-term word recall and word category association. [2]

AD8 Questionnaire: The "AD8" is a common phrase to refer to the Washington University Screening Test. It consists of eight basic questions which can be used by a primary care physician to assist in the determination if a loved one's issues are normal aging or are dementia. The clinician can ask the eight yes/no questions or can simply give it to the loved one on a clipboard to self-administer. If two or more of the questions are answered with a no, it indicates that the loved one may have dementia. [2] [3]

QDRS Test: The Quick Dementia Rating System is a ten-item questionnaire designed to be self-administered and only requires about five minutes. It covers ten areas and attempts to identify symptoms of Mild Cognitive Impairment, Alzheimer's Disease and non-Alzheimer's disorders including Lewy Body dementia, frontotemporal degeneration, vascular dementia plus other issues. This test was privately developed and copyrighted by James E. Galvin and New York University Langone Medical Center, New York, New York. [4] [5]

SAGE Test: This is the Self-Administered Geocognitive Examination. This test was developed by the Ohio State Werner Medical Center. It consists of a 15-question written exam using pencil and paper. Most of the questions should be answered correctly by a cognitively healthy person. The test will provide an excellent baseline for patients having cognitive decline. There are four different English language tests for administration at future visits. [6]

Clock Drawing Test: In this test, the administrator takes a piece of 8 ½ x 11 blank paper and draws a large circle on it with a pen. It is given to the person being tested with the instructions to draw a clock, first putting all the numbers on it and then showing a time. The administrator does not give any additional instructions. The test is a pass-fail. Cognitively healthy individuals should pass with ease. The clock-drawing test errors are:

1. Refusal to take the test
2. Missing numbers. All twelve should be shown in the correct locations
3. Missing hands
4. Wrong time shown
5. Numbers are repeated on the clock face
6. Numbers were substituted with another symbol.[7]

Mini-Cog Test: The mini-cognitive test is copyrighted by Soo Borson. It is simple and consists of only three steps:

Step 1: Three-word retention. The administrator looks directly at the person being tested and says, "Please listen carefully. I am going to say three words that I want you to repeat back to me and try to remember. The words are: banana, sunrise, chair." Of course, any three non-associated words can be used.

Step2: The clock drawing test. The administrator uses the same procedure as above.

Step 3: Three-word recall. After the clock drawing is completed, ask the person to recall the three words you stated in step one. The administrator then asks, "What were the three words I asked you to remember?"

The test is scored giving zero to three points for the three words and zero or two points for the clock drawing. If the clock drawing is perfect, give two points. If imperfect, give zero points. A perfect score is five. Any score of three points or less should prompt additional evaluation efforts to more accurately determine the individual's cognitive base line. [8]

Folstein MMSE Test: This test is the Mini Mental State Examination. It was developed in Canada by the British Columbia Ministry of Health. The test is a written 30-point questionnaire like the SAGE questionnaire. Most of the questions should be answered correctly by a cognitively healthy person. The test will provide an excellent baseline for patients having cognitive decline. Scores of 24-30 are considered normal, 19-23 are considered borderline and less than 19 are considered as cognitively impaired. [9]

ADAS-Cog Test: This test is the Alzheimer's disease assessment scale-cognitive subscale. There are various versions which measure memory, language, orientation and other cognitive abilities. It is much more extensive than the Mini-Cog and the MMSE tests. [10]

Addenbrooke's Cognitive Examination [ACE-R]: This is a test developed at Addenbrooke's Hospital, Cambridge, England and is available from the website of St. Vincent's University Hospital in Ireland. It is a brief neuropsychological assessment of cognitive functions and basically is an expansion of the MMSE. It is widely used to determine if a person has mild cognitive impairment and dementia. It measures attention, verbal fluency, language, memory, visuospatial ability and orientation to time and place. [11]

Addenbrooke's Cognitive Examination or ACE-III is a modification of the ACE-R test and was developed as a compromise following discussions with the Psychological Assessment Resources, Inc. firm who believed the ACE-R infringed on their copyright and commercial use. [12]

TYM Test: The Test Your Memory (TYM) Test is a short, self-administered test developed at Addenbrooke's Hospital, Cambridge, England. TYM is completed by patients themselves and involves ten tasks: Orientation, ability to copy a sentence, semantic knowledge about common facts, objects and meanings of words, calculation, verbal fluency similarities, naming, visuospatial abilities and recall of a previously copied sentence. [13]

GPCOG Interview: The General Practitioner Assessment of Cognition (GPCOG) test was developed in Australia and is a six-item interview designed to differentiate normal aging from dementia. It is very basic and starts with the administrator providing the person with a name and address. Then the person is asked for today's date. This is followed by the clock drawing test and then the subject is asked to tell the administrator what was reported in the news recently. Sufficiently distracted, the person is then asked to provide the name and address previously provided at the beginning. [14]

IQCODE Short Form: The Informant Questionnaire on Cognitive Decline in the Elderly Short Form was developed at the Australian National University. There is no copyright on the Short IQCODE form, so I am providing the 16 questions it addresses:

1. Remembering things about family and friends e.g. occupations, birthdays, addresses
2. Remembering things that have happened recently
3. Recalling conversations a few days later
4. Remembering his/her address and telephone number
5. Remembering what day and month it is
6. Remembering where things are usually kept
7. Remembering where to find things which have been put in a different place from usual
8. Knowing how to work familiar machines around the house
9. Learning to use a new gadget or machine around the house
10. Learning new things in general
11. Following a story in a book or on TV
12. Making decisions on everyday matters
13. Handling money for shopping
14. Handling financial matters e.g. the pension, dealing with the bank
15. Handling other everyday arithmetic problems e.g.

knowing how much food to buy, knowing how long between visits from family or friends
16. Using his/her intelligence to understand what's going on and to reason things through.

Then the form asks, for each question compared to ten years ago, was the loved one: much improved, a bit improved, not much change, a bit worse or much worse. [15]

Global Deterioration Scale (GDS): Developed by Dr. Barry Reisberg, this test summarizes a seven-level cognitive decline progression. The first through the fourth levels describe decline up to the mild stage of dementia:

- Level one: No cognitive decline
- Level two: Age Associated Memory Impairment
- Level three: Mild Cognitive Impairment
- Level four: Mild Dementia [16]

What Worked for Us That May Work for You

- Laura refused to take these tests, but it was a simple matter to ask a few of the questions on these tests every day in normal conversation and eventually determined her level of basic cognition
- I thoroughly researched the Internet until I was in my comfort zone about Laura's eventual diagnosis. This permitted me to address my efforts into practical matters that would help improve her quality of life
- Since Laura clearly understood dementia and its progression from being in close contact with her mother and sister who had progressed down the dementia slippery slope, I supported her wish to avoid thinking about the disease and to stay in denial as much as possible

- We both did our best to follow our doctor's advice to enjoy each day to the maximum

Positive Affirmations

"Success is liking yourself, liking what you do, and liking how you do it." – *Maya Angelou*

"When one door of happiness closes, another opens, but often we look so long at the closed door that we do not see the one that has been opened for us." – *Helen Keller*

"Courage and perseverance have a magical talisman, before which difficulties disappear and obstacles vanish into air." – *John Quincy Adams*

End Notes

[1]   https://www.alz.org/media/Documents/10-signs-worksheet
[2]   https://www.alz.org/media/Documents/ad8-dementia
[3]   https://www.consultgen.org/try-this/dementia/issue
[4]   James E. Galvin and New York University Langone Medical Center, New York New York. Copyrighted 2013.
[5]   https://www.ncbi.nlm.nih.gov/pmc/articles/PMC4
[6]   https://www.wexnermedical.osu.edu/brain
[7]   https://www. watermark.silverchair.com
[8]   https://www.mini-cog.com
[9]   https://www.ncbi.nlm.nih.gov/projects/gap/cgi
[10] https://www.ncbi.nih.gov/pmc/articles/pmc3873
[11] https://www.ipa-online.org/news-and-issues/add
[12] https://www.ncbi.nlm.nih.gov/pmc/articles/PMC6
[13] https://www.neurologyspecialists.org/registration
[14] https://www.gpcog.com.au
[15] https://www.cochranelibrary.com/cdsr/doi/10.1
[16] https://www.ncbi.nlm.nih.gov/pubmed/7114305

CHAPTER 13

The Right to Avoid a Dementia Diagnosis

"Wisdom is knowledge that is guided by understanding; we have to have the wisdom and the knowledge to understand why certain things happen in our lives and trust that God will lead us over any obstacles that comes in our way."
– Anonymous

We consciously chose to avoid obtaining a dementia diagnosis during Laura's mild stage. Why would we ever make that choice? What were we thinking? Did we ever regret making that decision? Is it morally ethical to do that? Was that an intelligent option? Laura and I were not experts in this area of life, but we were not rookies either. Memories of many loved ones living with dementia ran through our minds like movies. We could both easily and vividly recall and re-live these past personal experiences with loved ones who lived with dementia.

Here are several stories that detail the amount of experience we had with loved ones living with dementia. I clearly remember the first time Laura's mother did not recognize me, although I had been in her family for over three decades. We were visiting her farm home several hours from our home and as I sat in the living room reading a book, her mother walked in and asked who I was and what was I doing inside her home. At that time, Laura was using our car to visit her friends in the area, so after I explained the situation, I moved to the front porch rocker to make her feel safer with me out of her home. A few years later, she was admitted into a nursing home for care.

We helped Laura's older brother access medical care several times. On the last occasion, I was driving him and our wives back to his home after he received a medical procedure requiring hospitalization. His surgeon released him because he was cognitively normal. Laura and her sister in law were in the rear seat. I was driving our car and the brother was in the front passenger seat. About halfway to his home, I realized that he didn't know who I was and what we were doing. He seemed to be in complete confusion. I then drove to the nearest hospital where he was admitted and treated for a severe stroke, possibly due to a blood clot broken loose as a result of his recent surgery. Hospitals can be dangerous places.

Laura's oldest sister was a high-level special needs individual. She lived on the farm with her parents for her entire life until she was eventually admitted into a nursing home for care. When we took her out for visits, we learned her visual-spatial defects were advanced. She could not safely navigate curbs, steps and stairs by herself. She eventually also did not recognize us.

My father was housebound and bedbound due to strokes at the end of his life. My mother nursed him at home during those years. During his final year, he did not recognize me when I visited.

Laura had two aunts who lived with dementia at the end of their lives. One lived at home and one in a nursing home. They did not recognize who we were on our periodic visits.

On one visit to Laura's hometown, we visited a married couple who both were high school classmates. It was a nice, friendly visit until I asked for their telephone number so Laura could call them periodically. I then realized that neither one knew their number nor could either find it. This resulted in both becoming agitated, so we soon departed. Sometime later, both were admitted to nursing homes.

Laura's oldest brother had Parkinson's disease, lived at home and had a mother-daughter team provide 24x7 care during his last years. I could not tell if he recognized us on our visits because his medication seemed to keep him drowsy continuously and conversing was almost impossible.

Laura's next older sister lived in the same state as we did, about a half-day drive away. We visited her every three to four months for decades. After her husband died, she lived with her family members. During her last year, she lived in a nursing home and no longer recognized us when we visited.

Our experiences visiting loved ones in nursing homes versus living in their own homes with caregivers convinced us that, if we ever had to live with dementia, our preference was to live at home as long as possible.

Did we discuss dementia? Yes, but each time I referred to a loved one who had the disease, the memories were so painful for Laura that her eyes would tear up. I found it was easier on both of us to keep dementia conversations focused on the positive aspects of the loved ones who lived in their homes.

My protective and caring instinct came to the forefront. I worried that shedding light on this area of health would set in motion a sense of hopelessness for Laura. I did not want to cause her emotional stress nor have her feel she was a burden to me.

So Why Bother with a Diagnosis?

Laura knew she had dementia. I knew she had dementia. We were aware that Laura had a cognitive health issue. We both knowingly chose to avoid getting a formal medical diagnosis for numerous and, what we believed were valid, reasons. I know that I would not want to learn that I had an incurable dementia disease. This was Laura's choice and I supported it. I believe it is morally correct that a person can completely understand they have the disease and also make a competent and informed choice to not receive a diagnosis to confirm it.

The most important benefit of a diagnosis is to rule out reversible and treatable causes of dementia. I made certain our primary care doctor was aware of Laura's condition and monitored his many attempts over a several year period to find a treatable issue.

Naturally, I included Laura in the decision to be diagnosed or not. It is only common sense to allow the loved one living with dementia to decide whether they want to know or do not want to know if they positively, absolutely have dementia disease. Laura clearly not only did not want to know, but she willingly, consciously, and proactively avoided taking any action toward receiving a dementia assessment diagnosis.

Showtimers

I have personally witnessed many Oscar-worthy performances and Laura was always the star actress in each performance.

The stage for the healthcare Academy Award performances was set in our doctor's office when Laura and I visited for our routine six-month medical checkups. Our primary medical provider served us for decades and we both liked him. Naturally, we scheduled our appointments at the same time and entered the examination room together, since I have always been responsible for insurance paperwork and medication prescriptions.

Laura always wanted to bathe before the appointments. She applied her Chanel bath powder, moisturized her skin, dressed well and was perfectly groomed before leaving for the six-month doctor checkup. She knew to look her best before an important performance.

I checked us both in after we arrived at the reception desk. At that time, I usually provided a short, written summary of my observations of Laura in a sealed envelope with the doctor's name on it and this note: "Contents private: to be reviewed by the doctor before the examination of Laura." That way, the doctor was familiar with the current symptoms prior to our face-to-face appointment. Laura hated criticism. She felt that openly discussing her symptoms with anyone was admitting she was no longer a healthy woman. Since she would be embarrassed if I verbally covered this information with our clinician in his presence, I provided it in advance as a neat, clear summary. It worked for us.

After we walked into the examination room, it was show time! Laura turned on her charm and outgoing personality, asking the doctor about his wife, children and lovely home. She got the doctor to talk about his mother's health, his children's accomplishments and his family's recent vacations. During the examination, Laura rose to performance excellence in her actress role, attempting to distract the doctor to defeat any suggestions he had for a memory test or evaluation. Possible referrals to other specialists were also summarily rejected with artful verbal dodging. Using expert distraction, Laura always professed that she was in great health and ready for another foreign vacation trip. By the time we left, the doctor smiled and advised that he envied our vacation trips to Europe.

Dementia? Hell no! Laura was completely normal. Ask her. She told me numerous times that it was a waste of her time going to these six-month check-ups. Our physician's routine was to ask the same question twice to check short-term memory. Laura was aware of this trick; watched out for it and told the doctor he must be slipping because she had already answered that question.

Let me repeat this because it's that important: Laura knew she had dementia. I knew she had dementia. Our doctor knew she had dementia. We saw him every six months for routine appointments for years. He usually tried to make a referral to a specialist. We agreed to disagree on the need to visit a specialist and never consulted one. This was our choice, but most other people make the opposite choice as they are highly motivated to utilize specialists.

Laura believed she was fooling the doctor, but I knew he simply accepted that nothing could be done to help her. He did order numerous additional blood tests to rule out various possible physical causes of her dementia symptoms. He also gave her a through physical examination. Since Laura was physically healthy, there was little the doctor could do. Of course, on the way out the door, the doctor would mention that he had written a referral for Laura to see a specialist in neurology. When we stopped by the appointment desk, Laura would reach out and hold my hand. When the scheduling person gave us alternatives for the referral, Laura would squeeze my hand in her vice-like grip. This was her way to silently but clearly communicate that I better not agree to a specialist referral. Naturally, I understood the message and advised the scheduler that I would call back after I was home and reviewed our calendar. Laura would then relax her grip and smugly smile meaning that she believed she had defeated the medical establishment once again. There was no question that she performed this subterfuge to rationalize her deteriorating cognitive abilities and thus minimize her fears of the future. I felt that I would be heartless if I escalated this issue, so I accepted our decision to evade confrontation with medical specialists.

On the trip home, we discussed the visit and the possible referrals Laura rejected. She dismissed each issue by saying, "These doctors only want our money. I don't need any more tests or doctor visits. They always make us wait. First, we wait in the reception room, then we wait in the doctor's office. It's too much trouble and too expensive. There's nothing wrong with me. Our business is our business. I don't want everyone to know our business. You better not tell anyone our business!"

Laura was the boss and I was the complicit accomplice. So, we both were united in avoiding a dementia diagnosis. Was it the right or the wrong approach? Each caregiver decision-maker will have to judge which strategy is correct in their case. What worked for us may not work for others.

Naturally, I felt guilty about my lack of success in getting Laura to obtain a baseline cognitive evaluation and to start the standard medications. So, in lieu of medications, I researched the Internet and became convinced that the specialized medications had little or no value in treating dementia. I spent hours reading about the value of possible alternative supplements. I tried several different supplements, but none seemed to have any positive benefit. I learned about baseline cognitive evaluations and could estimate Laura's scores from my daily observations of her behavior.

I rationalized my complicity in our joint subterfuge by ensuing Laura took her daily routine medications and supplements, had a healthy diet, got daily exercise by walking during shopping outings and had extra socialization with friends and family. We visited our grandsons almost daily after they arrived home from school. They were always happy to see us because we brought their favorite fast food sandwich treat. These were happy days for Laura.

What Worked for Us That May Work for You

- I accepted that showtimers is a common behavior by loved ones living with dementia.
- I accepted that it is common for a loved one living with dementia to choose to avoid a dementia diagnosis.
- I learned the mechanics of the basic cognitive tests. They are relatively simple and readily available on the Internet. Using subterfuge, I tested Laura by asking a few questions every day.
- After completing the cognitive test questions, I was aware of the rough score and was able to communicate the initial baseline to the doctor and then I reported the present status or degree of deterioration on future visits.
- I provided a short, written summary of Laura's status in a sealed envelope marked private before the doctor's examination by simply giving it to the receptionist upon initial arrival.
- On each medical visit, in all circumstances and in all conditions I never, ever discussed Laura's symptoms with the doctor in her presence. I believed this would be disrespectful, hurtful, cruel and highly counterproductive. I believe Laura would forget the words I'd said, but never forget how she felt after I said them.
- Laura thought she and I were playing a chess game about

doctor visits. Who was winning? Who was losing? Who knows? Who cares?

- Laura's intuition was extremely valuable and I listened carefully when she expressed it.
- I found that not initiating any approved drugs for early stage dementia had the wonderful benefits of avoiding a host of possible unpleasant side effects for Laura.
- I supported avoiding a dementia diagnosis as a beneficial strategy because there was no known or possible cure, treatment, reduction, remission or benefit from initiating drug treatment.
- Alternative, complimentary, non-drug approaches are generally believed to moderate the symptoms. I took the initiative to increase our physical exercise, mental exercise and social activities.
- For some people, the diagnosis of dementia can come as a relief, as they now know exactly what is the cause of their problem. That was not our case. We both believed that dementia was simply a part of life that occurred to about everyone in Laura's family when they became aged. We believed dementia was something to accept and live with using the best of our abilities.
- We did not battle dementia nor did we struggle against it. Why bother? It is an incurable disease that occurs near the end of a person's life.
- I believed both Laura and I had a limited time on earth which made the importance of a good quality of life for each minute, each hour and each day for us being of paramount importance. This was our goal and we pursued it.

What is the value of a dementia diagnosis if the loved one is never told?

Worldwide, in high income countries, only 50 percent of people living with dementia receive a formal diagnosis. In low and middle-income countries, less than 10 percent of people living with dementia are diagnosed. [1]

In our country, clinicians must overcome their reluctance of providing a dementia diagnosis to the loved one living with it. One study concluded that only about half of primary care physicians ever tell their patients they have Alzheimer's. [1, 2, 3, 4]

One major reason for reluctance on the part of a primary care doctor to diagnose dementia in the early stage is the reality that it is difficult to differentiate between early dementia and Mild Cognitive Impairment (MCI). If the patient has MCI but not dementia an important ethical dilemma exists. Since some MCI progresses to dementia and some does not, the decision to inform the patient that maybe they will have dementia in the future is gut-wrenching for the doctor. Uncertainty about an increased risk is a very real and difficult issue. If the doctor errs on the side of advising that there is a high potential for eventual dementia, then the loved one may experience feelings of hopelessness and grief unnecessarily. If the doctor errs on the side of advising that there is minimal risk for eventual dementia, then the loved one may choose to avoid confronting important future legal, care and financial planning.

Another study showed that most geriatric psychiatrists rarely or only sometimes informed patients of their diagnosis of dementia. [5, 6]

A report released by the Alzheimer's Association stated that, among those suffering with Alzheimer's disease, just 45 percent of people are informed of their diagnosis by their doctor. That figure includes caregivers as well. When the data excluded information only shared with caregivers, the disclosure rate dropped to 33 percent. Most caregivers are generally reluctant to confront their loved one and tell them of the diagnosis when they initially learn of it. [3, 4]

The U.S. government has set a goal of increasing the percentage of patients and caregivers who have been informed of their Alzheimer's diagnosis (the government only tracks this form of dementia), from 34.8 percent to 38.3 percent by the year 2020. [3, 4] In round numbers, this means that, in reality, only about one in three people living with dementia are ever furnished a diagnosis that they have a dementia disease. The other two are never told. They may be the lucky ones!

Other factors impact this issue. Sometimes the disease progresses so fast that a loved one loses competence to understand the diagnosis. If so, then informing the loved one about the diagnosis becomes a non-issue. For those in the moderate and severe stage of dementia, only 13 percent and 6 percent, respectively, of physicians discussed the diagnosis with their patient. [1, 2]

Also, some families believe that it is important to keep the loved one in the dark to spare them the mental and emotional suffering from that knowledge. Several studies of Asian-American cultures have found this to be their norm. [7] Naturally, some primary medical practitioners believe that the diagnosis should be made by a specialist following an extensive examination and that specialist is the best person to provide the diagnosis. You could call this passing the buck or you could call this using good judgment or both.

Okay, for those who do choose to be diagnosed and are officially informed, one in four with dementia then choose to hide or conceal their diagnosis. Why? They believe they may become stigmatized and therefore excluded from everyday life. They want to be treated as a normal, healthy person with emphasis on their abilities and not on their deficits. [8]

When the diagnosis is understood, the loved one living with dementia can make important decisions and plans regarding their future. Legal, care and financial matters can be clearly addressed and optimum choices made. Designating a financial power of attorney, medical power of attorney and preparing a living will are only a few of the priorities to be considered. Naturally, the loved one needs to have legal capacity at the time these decisions are made. In our case, we handled these issues early in the process and didn't need a diagnosis to motivate us to take common and logical legal actions.

Dementia trials exist in almost every major medical center and large municipality. Naturally, trials require the participant to personally agree. Neither of us wanted to do the paperwork or devote time to a clinical trial. To my knowledge, of the millions of world-wide clinical trials involving dementia, very few have resulted in positive benefits. Also, since we chose to not utilize any approved dementia medications due to potential negative side-effects, we did not want to test new medications. Due to repeated drug trial failures, many large pharmaceutical companies have chosen to discontinue their initiatives to find new dementia drugs.

It is believed that the approved medications are more likely to be helpful when used in the early stage. Although they cannot cure or reverse the disease, they are believed to result in maintaining a person's current level of function. Since they cannot cure or reverse dementia, why bother with medications? Some of these medications have serious negative side effects for some people.

Caregivers who do support using the approved medications should be aware that the most important guideline is to start low and go slow. Observe how your loved one responds to the lowest dose of the new medication and, if their reaction is positive, then maintain that low initial dosage or, when increases are required, smaller is better.

Positive Affirmations

"Anything in life that we don't accept will simply make trouble for us until we make peace with it." – *Shakti Gawain*

"We can have peace if we let go of wanting to change the past and wanting to control the future." – *Lester Levinson*

"If you have the guts to keep making mistakes, your wisdom and intelligence leap forward with huge momentum." – *Holly Near*

"I learned that courage was not the absence of fear, but the triumph over it. The brave man is not he who does not feel afraid, but he who conquers that fear." – *Nelson Mandela*

"Faith gives us strength and reassurance and leaves us bathed in the wisdom that we are never alone." – *Debbie Ford*

End Notes

[1]   BMC Health Services Research 18, 29 November 2018: 910 (2018)
      https://www.bmchealthservres.biomedcentral.com

[2]   Western Journal of Medicine, 2000, Nov; 173(5); 318-323
      https://www.ncbi.nlm.nih.gov/pmc/articles/PMC10

[3]   Kimberly Leonard, US News Magazine, March 24, 2015, "Most Alzheimer's Patients Not Told About Their Diagnosis."
      https://www.usnews.com/news/articles/2015/03/

[4]   2018 Alzheimer's Disease Facts and Figures Report – Alzheimer's Association. Study conducted by the Rush Alzheimer's Disease Center and the Rush Institute for Healthy Aging in Chicago, IL and funded by the National Institute for Aging (NIA).
      https://www.alz.org/media/Documents/facts-and-figures

[5]   Kathleen Allen, LCSW, C-ASWCM, Senior Care Management Service, LLC, October 25, 2017.
      https://www.brightfocus.org/alzheimers/article/informing

[6]   Alayna Jaques, Population Health Learning Network, Annals of Long-Term Care newsletter, February 28, 2014. Reference 3: Rice et.al. Breaking the bad news: what do psychiatrist tell patients with dementia about their illness. Int J Geriatric Psychiatry 1994:467-471. https://www.managementhealth-careconnect.com/

[7]   Journal of Cross-Cultural Gerontology. 2018 Sep: 23(3): 283-299
      https://www.ncbi.nim.nih.gov

[8]   Culture Change Network of Georgia posted January 15, 2019
      https://www.culturechangega.org

CHAPTER 14

The Right to Obtain an Accurate Dementia Diagnosis

"You have to accept whatever comes and the only important thing is that you meet it with courage and with the best you have to give."
– Eleanor Roosevelt

Yes, the title of this chapter is correct. You have the right to obtain an accurate diagnosis of which dementia disease your loved one is experiencing. Why would you even need this, right? Why is it called an accurate diagnosis as opposed to something else? No one would want an inaccurate diagnosis! Can't every doctor tell when someone has a dementia disease? Are not most dementias Alzheimer's? What is the problem?

This may be the most important chapter of this book. It also may be the most informative. Does it read like a textbook? Yes, but you will find it much more interesting this way. However, it definitely is technical and sometimes boring. So, if you currently have minimal interest in obtaining an accurate diagnosis, then feel free to only scan this material. But make a mental note that, if and when you have the need to obtain an accurate diagnosis, you will know where to review the basics as your loved one undergoes the diagnostic process. You will learn what you need to know to serve as a competent advocate for your loved one.

Yes, if you wish to search your local library, bookstores and the

Internet, you can eventually learn everything I cover in this chapter. I may be biased, but I feel this chapter covers the diagnosis subject much more thoroughly than other treatments that are available. You will learn that a diagnosis of dementia for your loved one is almost certain to be nearly 100 per cent accurate, but an accurate diagnosis of the type of dementia is at best 80 percent accurate. Does it matter so much? Unfortunately, it does. That is why I feel this is the most important chapter of this book.

Laura chose to avoid obtaining a dementia diagnosis in the mild stage. Even if she had, it would not have been accurate. How do I know that? Well, when she was eventually diagnosed late in the moderate stage, her diagnosis was not even accurate then! So, isn't dementia just dementia? No, it isn't!

In Laura's case, she had mixed dementia. It consisted of Alzheimer's disease, vascular disease and Lewy Body disease. The Lewy Body component was not recognized until she had a major adverse side effect to a medication that is wrong for loved ones with Lewy Body dementia. The hospital prescribed a common anti-psychotic medication which almost killed her. This happened even though she was hospitalized at the time and was being monitored continually by vital sign medical apparatus. Additionally, they had an attendant stationed just outside her room on a 24/7 basis to prevent her from wandering. Her care was continually supervised electronically by nurses and she was periodically attended by hospital physicians.

But that's a story for a future book when I address the moderate dementia stage. In that book, I will address Laura's dementia diagnosis and our very stressful hospitalization experiences. In this book, you will learn that you have the right to obtain an accurate dementia disease diagnosis. You will learn there are difficult roadblocks that will have to be faced by the loved one and the caregiver. You will discover that the process is burdensome, time intensive, costly and emotionally charged.

The reason that obtaining an accurate diagnosis is difficult is because the complexity of an accurate diagnosis is immense.

Here is my experience and review of readily available information on this subject. This information comes from https://www.
aaicmedia@alz.org:

1. Primary health care physicians are handicapped by the
   minimal diagnostic procedures they can employ. Thankfully,
   Medicare rules were changed in 2018 to pay clinicians for a
   basic screening during the annual wellness visit to evaluate
   possible cognitive impairments. At best, this basic screening
   can result in a referral to a specialist.
2. Specialists are limited by the diagnostic procedures the insurance industry will approve. The more advanced diagnostic
   procedures are very costly and the health insurance industry
   sometimes balks at covering some needed but expensive tests.

Progress to improve the diagnosis of dementia is slow but is be-
ing made. Here are a few excerpts from a press release from the
Alzheimer's Association International Conference (AAIC) held in
Chicago during July 2018:

> "Despite more than two decades of advances in diagnostic
> criteria and technology, symptoms of Alzheimer's disease
> and Related Dementias (ADRD) too often go unrecognized
> or are misattributed, causing delays in appropriate diagno-
> ses and care that are both harmful and costly. Contributing
> to the variability and inefficiency is the lack of multidisci-
> plinary ADRD evaluation guidelines to inform U.S. clinicians
> in primary and specialty care settings."

> "... There are currently no U.S. national consensus best clini-
> cal practice guidelines that provide integrated multispecialty
> recommendations for the clinical evaluation of cognitive im-
> pairment suspected to be due to ADRD for use by primary
> and specialty care medical and nursing practitioners."

However, an AAIC workgroup is addressing this issue and their preliminary recommendations include:

1. "All middle-aged or older individuals who self-report or whose care partner or clinician report cognitive, behavioral or functional changes should undergo a timely evaluation."
2. "Concerns should not be dismissed as 'normal aging' without a proper assessment."
3. "Evaluation should involve not only the patient and clinician but, almost always, involve a care partner (e.g., family member or confidant)."

Taking a step toward a "U.S. national consensus best clinical practice guideline," the AAIC workgroup responsible for this subject issued a Clinical Practice Guideline (CPG) consisting of 20 consensus recommendations in July 2018. Here is a summary of the 20 AAIC consensus recommendations in layman's terms:

There are four general recommendations for the primary care clinician:

1. Initiate a multi-tiered evaluation including patient history, lab tests, standard cognitive office tests and the like.
2. If the evaluation shows rapidly progressing dementia, the clinician should strongly consider referral to a specialist.
3. The various types of assessment tiers and tests used should be based on the individual.
4. Establish a collaborative dialogue with the patient and care partner to educate, communicate, inform and ensure ongoing management, care and support.

There are two recommendations for the primary care clinician taking the history of the present illness:

5. The evaluation should include patient cognition, activities of daily living, mood and other neuropsychiatric symptoms and sensory and motor function.
6. Ensure the cognitive-behavioral symptoms being evaluated result in reliable, specific and individualized information.

There are four recommendations concerning office-based examination accomplished by the primary care clinician and the specialist clinician:

7. Perform an examination of cognition, mood and behavior (mental status exam) and a dementia-focused neurological examination.
8. Use validated tools to evaluate cognitive-behavioral symptoms.
9. In cases of diagnostic uncertainty, the patient should be referred to a specialist.
10. A specialist should perform a comprehensive history and office-based examination of cognitive, neuropsychiatric and neurological functions.

There is one recommendation for the neuropsychological evaluation:

11. When office-based cognitive assessment is not sufficient, then neuropsychological testing of learning, memory, executive function, visuospatial function and language should be accomplished.

Laboratory and imaging tests have seven recommendations:

12. Standard blood and urine tests should be obtained.
13. Magnetic resonance imaging (MRI) of the brain should be obtained. If an MRI is not available, a computed tomography (CT) of the brain should be obtained.

14. Additional laboratory tests should be obtained based on the individual patient.
15. If diagnostic uncertainty still exists, molecular imaging using an FDG-PET scan of the brain should be obtained. The abbreviations stand for fluorodeoxyglucose-positron emission tomography.
16. If diagnostic uncertainty still exists, a cerebrospinal fluid (CSF) sample should be considered and may be obtained.
17. If diagnostic uncertainty still exists, an amyloid positron emission tomography (PET) scan should be considered and may be obtained.
18. If the patient has a family history of dementia, genetic testing should be considered and conducted if warranted.

Communication of diagnostic findings and follow-up has two recommendations:

19. Throughout the evaluation process, a dialogue should be maintained with the patient and the care partner to ensure an understanding and appreciation of the presence and severity of the dementia.
20. In communicating findings to the patient and care partner, the clinician should honestly and compassionately inform them of the name, characteristics, severity and stage of the disease. Also, the clinician should advise future expectations, treatment options, safety considerations, support services and care planning. [1]

Additionally, based on my experience and my review of available information on this subject, getting an exact, accurate diagnosis also faces the following complexity:

1. The earliest symptoms can occur to affect any brain function: Memory, language, visuospatial perception, behavior

or motor function. The brain region affected corresponds to the symptoms so a lay person would tend to believe an accurate diagnosis can be made as soon as the loved one's unique symptom(s) are identified. Yes, clinicians can usually verify that a person has dementia with a high degree of accuracy. There is no problem with the accuracy of the general diagnosis of dementia. However, once the general diagnosis is made, then determining the specific type of dementia is extremely difficult and/or nearly impossible in the mild or early stage.

2. Sometimes the symptoms are caused by more than one dementia disease and/or sometimes a loved one has dementia plus other co-existing physical issues. The symptoms and brain changes associated with several different dementia and physical diseases can and do overlap. This is difficult to explain to others and can be stressful for the loved one living with dementia.

3. Due to the diverse types of dementia, the early warning signs come in a wide spectrum of symptoms. In the mild stage, the symptoms vary depending on the different type of dementia being experienced. The diagnosis of dementia is based on a process of elimination. A host of physical issues can cause dementia-like symptoms and each possibility has to be ruled out before a dementia disease diagnosis can be made.

4. There is no absolute set of symptoms to guide the progression from normal aging to dementia. However, there are many early symptoms that can be easily recognized and used as indicators that a physician should be consulted.

5. The medical community firmly believes that timely treatment will result in moderating the symptoms and, thereby, improve the quality of life for a person living with dementia. Although the medical community sometimes seems to stress the importance of prescription drugs for treatment of the various symptoms of dementia, some experts in this field believe the benefits of a person-centered, non-pharmacological approach may exceed the value of medications.

6. Taking away an individual's driving privileges is extremely difficult.

7. The complexity of a diagnosed dementia disease in the mild stage is compounded by the stigma attached to all mental illnesses by society.

8. When dementia is formally confirmed by a diagnosis, long-term care insurance usually cannot be obtained.

9. Usually the assets of both spouses must be spent down to the point where they are nearly impoverished for State aid to step in and care for the ill spouse. Transferring assets to others to qualify for governmental assistance is not possible nor advisable due to what is called "asset look back" periods required by state laws. An elder care attorney who specializes in this area may provide accurate and beneficial advice to aid in making optimum financial and legal decisions.

10. Amyloid positron emission tomography (PET) scans are not routinely used to confirm an Alzheimer's diagnosis because these amyloid PET brain imaging scans are not currently paid for by Medicare. The rationale is that, since Alzheimer's disease is incurable, getting the scan would not change the course of the disease or of the treatment. In addition, secondary health insurance plans which normally pay a benefit after Medicare does, also do not currently pay for this type of test due to the same reason. [2]

How many of the original Alzheimer's diagnosis cases are correct, incorrect or just flat out wrong? There is a large-scale study in progress as of this writing. The preliminary results show that about one-third of the participants had their cognitive impairment diagnosis altered based on the results of amyloid PET imaging. In almost two-thirds of the cases, clinicians changed their specific recommendation for participants including the use of medications and counseling. In about one in three cases, participants who had been previously diagnosed with Alzheimer's were able to rule out that disease based on a lack of amyloid buildup. In some cases, a non-Alzheimer dementia disease caused their symptoms. In other cases, evaluations of alternative and possible reversible causes such as medication side effects, sleep disorders or depression could then be properly addressed. Also, many of the participants who had not been previously diagnosed with Alzheimer's received a new diagnosis based on the PET scan. [2]

When an Alzheimer's diagnosis is made, clinicians or specialists do not say it is Alzheimer's disease. Rather, they say it is "probable or possible Alzheimer's disease" and then state the qualification that this disease can only be identified accurately after death if a brain autopsy is conducted. But how many of the pathology findings are consistent with the previous diagnosis? In about 20 percent of those loved ones who previously had an Alzheimer's diagnosis, their brain autopsy showed they **did not** have the characteristic amyloid plaques associated with this disease. Unexpectedly, various studies ranging from 10 to 60 percent of individuals who were both cognitively normal during their lives and had a brain autopsy did have the characteristic amyloid plaques. [3]

To put a round number to this issue, expect a misdiagnosis rate of about 20 percent even by experienced clinicians using advanced diagnostic procedures. Lewy Body dementia (LBD) is misdiagnosed as Alzheimer's 29 percent of the time. Frontotemporal lobar degeneration (FTLD) has a 19 percent rate of being misdiagnosed as Alzheimer's. [4]

These difficulties have resulted in more and more diagnoses to be labeled mixed dementia. The most common mixed dementia diagnoses are Alzheimer's and vascular dementia, Alzheimer's and Lewy Body dementia or all three: Alzheimer's, vascular dementia and Lewy Body dementia. [5]

Various large studies have found mixed dementia as low as 10 percent and one small study found it as high as 50 percent. [5, 6] A large post mortem pathology study found that more than 50 percent of Alzheimer's cases had coexisting pathology in addition to the hallmark Alzheimer's brain changes. The most common was vascular issues and the second most common was Lewy bodies. [6]

Laura had mixed dementia: Alzheimer's, vascular dementia, and Lewy Body dementia. In my opinion, the majority of all dementias are mixed dementia.

So how does a caregiver go about obtaining an accurate diagnosis for their loved one?

First, do your homework. Caregivers and family members are essential to the process of diagnosing mild or early-stage Alzheimer's disease or other dementias. There is no question in my mind that the caregiver being closely involved with clinician visits is of paramount importance. The caregiver should do necessary homework. Learn as much as possible about dementia. Become more familiar with the do-it-yourself diagnosis chapter and through either willing assistance or subterfuge, complete several of these self-measurement evaluations in the comfort of your home. Review and mark up the signs and symptoms chapter of this book to record your loved one's dementia symptoms. You will then be better prepared to summarize this information when you and your loved one are interviewed by your primary care physician.

The caregiver should be prepared to furnish input during the visit by documenting notes of their observations involving changes in their loved one's mood, anxiety, sleep, personality and interpersonal relationships. Behavioral symptoms sometimes appear in advance of cognitive symptoms involving memory and thinking. The caregiver is the best source to validate or deny the loved one's own input.

Continue to periodically review the chapters earlier in this book that cover the cognitive, physical and emotional symptoms. When referred to a specialist, the caregiver should be knowledgeable and have the ability to communicate the loved one's symptoms in more detail.

Second, meet with your doctor. Start with your Primary Medical Physician, also called a primary medical provider or primary care physician [PCP]. Sometimes, this primary doctor is called the family doctor, internist, general internist or doctor of internal medicine, nurse practitioner or physician's assistant. Although the loved one may be referred to various specialists, this primary clinician is the person who will be providing care over the many years in the future. A one-on-one trusting relationship with this clinician is vital and critical.

The primary care clinician will take a complete medical history, perform a physical examination, order and review various laboratory tests and administer some short written cognitive tests. This clinician's objective is to rule out reversible, treatable and/or non-cognitive causes of the symptoms and to complete a thorough memory screening to evaluate if a referral to a specialist is necessary.

Laboratory tests ordered by your primary care clinician to rule out possible non-cognitive issues include blood and urine tests. Blood tests will test for infection, anemia, the body's electrolyte balance (salt and water), liver function, thyroid function, vitamin B12 deficiency, medication interactions and dosing problems. Urine tests will look for possible urinary or bladder infection.

Cognitive tests ordered by your primary care clinician are used to measure and evaluate memory, concentration, problem solving, counting and language skills. These tests will include both verbal and paper assessments. They could include the Mini-Mental State Examination (MMSE) which only takes about five minutes to complete. It assesses very basic skills including reading, writing, orientation and short-term memory. Three other basic screening tests recommended by the Alzheimer's Association for use during the Medicare Annual Wellness visit are the General Practitioner Assessment of Cognition (GPCOG), the Mini-Cognitive test (Mini-Cog) and the Memory Impairment Screen (MIS). They are all easy to administer and rapid to complete. [7]

Third, comply with referrals to specialists made by your primary medical physician. Accept that your clinician will make several referrals and that the referrals will take time and energy. Make a commitment to comply with all referral appointments. The loved one living with dementia may also be referred to a physical therapist for a gait and/or balance evaluation. [9]

Comprehensive Neurological Examination

The loved one living with dementia may be referred to a neurological specialist. If so, this examination is the gold standard for neurological evaluation. These are some of the things that may occur with one of these exams:

1. Written and verbal tests may include assessment of memory loss or forgetfulness; orientation to person, place, and time; decision making and problem-solving abilities; language skills such as speech comprehension, conversational skills and word finding; writing and reading abilities; functional independence regarding self-care activities of daily living; mood, behavioral and personality change; attention and concentration abilities. [7]

2. One common written test is the Alzheimer's Disease Assessment Scale-Cognitive (ADAS-Cog). It is more thorough than the MMSE and is also used for loved ones with mild symptoms. Drug trials and research studies often use this test to track their findings. [8]

3. The neurological team will use various laboratory tests, verbal and written cognitive tests, a physical examination, various advanced imaging scans and interviews. The end result will be a comprehensive evaluation of the loved one's memory, language skills, visual perception, ability to focus attention, movement, senses, balance, reflexes and other physical and cognitive abilities. A significant benefit of accomplishing the comprehensive neurological examination is to establish a base line to help monitor the progression of dementia. [9]

Structural vs. Functional Brain Imaging

Neurological imaging tests and scans may include **structural brain imaging**:

1. Magnetic resonance imaging (MRI) of the brain is a technology to accomplish structural imaging of the brain. The result highlights changes to certain affected areas. Information such as the shape and volume of brain tissue is obtained. Brains of people living with Alzheimer's disease shrink significantly as the disease progresses into the severe stage. The area of the brain with the most shrinkage is an indicator of which dementia disease is present. [9, 10]
2. Computerized tomography (CT) of the brain is a technology which involves taking many X-rays from different angles in a very short time. The results are then used to display a three-dimensional image of the brain. The CT test is used to rule out other possible causes of dementia like stroke, brain tumor or brain bleeding. [9, 10]
3. MRI procedures involve the use of very powerful magnets and radio waves to display a very clear three-dimensional image of the brain. It provides superior resolution and is currently generally considered the optimum radiological test of choice. It serves to both rule out non-cognitive but treatable causes of dementia and also to better determine the different types of dementia. [9, 10]

Neurological imaging tests and scans may also include **functional brain imaging** of the brain:

1. Positron emission tomography (PET), functional MRI (fMRI), Fluorodeoxyglucose-positron emission tomography (FDG-PET) and magnetoencephalography (MEG) are technologies which accomplish functional imaging of the brain. They highlight how well cells in various brain regions are functioning by showing how actively the cells use sugar or oxygen. [9, 10]
2. FDF-PET measures which regions of the brain have a reduced use of glucose. Reduced glucose metabolism in specific areas

is used to determine the cause of someone's symptoms and which type of dementia is being experienced. [9, 10]

Molecular Brain Imaging and Cerebrospinal Fluid Analysis

Neurological imaging tests and scans may also include **molecular brain imaging** of the brain:

Single photon emission computerized tomography (SPECT), PET and fMRI are technologies which accomplish molecular imaging of the brain. They use highly targeted radiotracers to determine cellular or chemical changes linked to specific dementias. PET imaging with the use of a certain radiotracer can detect amyloid plaques which are a possible indicator of Alzheimer's disease. Other radiotracers that bind to different chemicals in the brains are used to assist in the diagnosis of other types of dementia. [9, 10]

Neurological imaging tests and scans may also include **cerebrospinal fluid analysis:**

Cerebrospinal fluid (CSF) is a clear fluid that bathes and cushions the brain and spinal cord. A sample is taken from the lower spine to check for certain protein markers that could be the cause of the onset of dementia. [9, 10]

Various combinations of these specialized imaging and tests may be required as determined by the neurological team. Duke University researchers believe that combining the results of three tests will produce a high degree of diagnostic accuracy for Alzheimer's disease. They are the MRI, the FDG-PET and the CSP analysis. [11]

Comprehensive Neuropsychological Evaluation

A referral to a psychologist, psychiatrist, geriatric psychologist, geriatric psychiatrist, neuropsychologist or some other specialist trained in the diagnosis of the various dementia diseases may be made. If so, the mental health team can determine whether depression or some other mental health condition is causing the loved one's signs and symptoms. [12]

Diagnosis of Alzheimer's Disease

Remember that a diagnosis of definite Alzheimer's disease can be made only at the time of an autopsy because it requires examination of actual brain tissue. A diagnosis of early-stage or mild Alzheimer's disease usually falls into one of two categories:

1. **Probable Alzheimer's** which indicates the medical team has ruled out all other medical issues that may be causing the dementia. That is, no other problem or cause for dementia can be found. [13]
2. **Possible Alzheimer's** indicates the presence of another co-existing medical issue that could be causing the early stage evaluation of Alzheimer's disease. The loved one's disease process appears different from what is normally seen. That is, the dementia may have another cause. However, Alzheimer's disease is still considered the primary cause of the loved one's dementia symptoms. [13]

Positive Affirmations

"Caring about others, running the risk of feeling, and leaving an impact on people, brings happiness." – *Harold Kushner, Rabbi*

End Notes

[1]   AAIC, July 22, 2018, AADx-CPG workgroup, First Practice Guidelines for Clinical Evaluation of Alzheimer's disease and other dementias for Primary and Specialty Care. https://www.aaicmedia@alz.org
[2]   Journal of the American Medical Society (JAMA), April 2, 2019 https://www.ideas-study.org/2019/04/01/results-of-t
[3]   Journal of the American Medical Society (JAMA), May 19, 2015

https://www.jamanetwork.com/journals/jama/fullarticle

[4]   The Journal of the Alzheimer's Association. Accuracy of Clinical Diagnosis of Alzheimer's disease in Alzheimer's Disease Centers (ADCS).
https://www.alzheimersanddementia.com/article

[5]   Alzheimer's Society, UK, what is mixed dementia?
https://www.alzheimers.org.uk/blog/what-is-mixed-dementia

[6]   2018 Alzheimer's Disease Facts and Figures Report – Alzheimer's Association. Study conducted by the Rush Alzheimer's Disease Center and the Rush Institute for Healthy Aging in Chicago, IL and funded by the National Institute for Aging (NIA).
https://www.alz.org/media/Documents/facts-and-figures

[7]   Very Well Health newsletter; Ester Heerema, MSW, updated May 22, 2017.
https://www.verywellhealth.com/what-is-the-gpcog

[8]   Very Well Health newsletter; Ester Heerema, MSW, updated May 18, 2017.
https://www.verywellhealth.com/alzheimer

[9]   Stanford University Health Care
https://www.stanfordhealthcare.org/medical-condition

[10] Harvard University Health Help Guide
https://www.helpguide.org/harvard/recognizing-alzheimers

[11] Medical News Today, Christian Nordqvist, December 28, 2012.
https://www.medicalnewstoday.com/articles/254

[12] Mayo Clinic; Dementia; Diagnosis
http://www.mayoclinic.org/diseases-conditions

[13] National Institute on Aging, U.S. National Institute of Health.
https://www.nia.nih.gov/health/how-alzheimers-diagnosed

CHAPTER 15

Telling the Diagnosis

"For over 30 years, I've preached that out of pain comes joy, out of brokenness comes wholeness, and out of death comes new life. I am determined to live that now as I face the challenges of dementia."
– The Very Rev. Tracey Lind

Informing the Loved One of Their Dementia Diagnosis

The diagnosis is complete. It is time to inform your loved one. This is the hard part! This is the hard part because many elderly individuals fear dementia. Some would rather not be told they have an incurable illness that cannot even be slowed. Others may prefer to use the psychological crutch of denial.

Many people view advanced dementia as a humiliating disease negatively affecting physical, mental and emotional health. Some people fear the future loss of independence and competence. Others fear the potential loss of dignity and personality. Many people fear the stigma some people commonly associate with mental illnesses. Naturally outgoing people may fear becoming socially isolated. Some seriously depressed individuals may contemplate suicide after learning of the diagnosis. You are dealing with a powder keg! It is important to be cautious and facilitate the best delivery of this news. It may be the worst news your loved one has ever heard in their life.

When the loved one asks the caregiver questions and indicates a desire to know, the caregiver must remember he or she is not a physician. "I don't know" is an honest and correct answer. Do not speculate. Not knowing the exact diagnosis but speculating and informing the loved one that they may have an incurable, untreatable and fatal disease would be poor judgment and possibly cruel. The caregiver has probably never confronted this issue before and he or she does not have a basis of experience to utilize. Definitely avoid giving a direct answer. It may be best to say, "We will find out. Our doctors will get to the bottom of this and give us an answer." When the caregiver is certain that the loved one wants to know, then the diagnosis should be finalized and planning should begin so that the loved one can be told in a humane and compassionate manner.

Delivering a dementia diagnosis may be the most undesirable task a doctor ever performs. The medical community is trained to consider how, when, where and why to advise when a person has a disease. Your loved one's primary care physician or one of the specialists will typically take the lead on this issue. A major concern of the primary care physician is the loved one's risk of suicide. If the loved one has co-existing depression, then suicide prevention is an issue that will have to be addressed. Without co-existing major mental issues, then suicide risk is very minimal and may be discounted. Nevertheless, some clinicians fear the consequences of frank disclosure as much as the loved one fears being diagnosed. [1]

Also, put yourself in the clinician's place for a moment. He or she has a tough job. The clinician must be 100% certain that the symptoms, tests, imaging and examination actually prove that the loved one has a dementia disease. But how reliable are they? If so, exactly which specific type of dementia disease does the loved one have and what is the degree of certainty? If the clinician is not completely certain, how is that explained to the person receiving the diagnosis?

The primary care clinician is in the business of saving lives and helping people overcome illness. Naturally, he or she is reluctant to deliver the news that dementia diseases have no cure, cannot be slowed and are always fatal.

The clinician will have to advise what drugs are available to moderate the symptoms. But he or she knows that they have limited benefits. The clinician doesn't want to be criticized for prescribing drugs that may be ineffective and has to consider if the side effects will be worse than the dementia symptoms.

There are other important things to consider. For instance, is it unsafe to let the loved one continue to drive? Is it required that the doctor inform the local driving agency that the driver's license be revoked now or, if not now, when? Confronting the withdrawal of an individual's driving privileges is extremely difficult by the doctor and for the family.

The doctor knows that long term care insurance may be impossible to obtain after the diagnosis is delivered. The financial, physical and emotional burdens facing the family will be immense.

Thoughts About How To Proceed

Planning, staging and delivering the initial news of the diagnosis:

The final decision as to who is going to tell the loved one about his or her dementia diagnosis is not difficult. It is the clinician's responsibility. The medical profession is trained and qualified to tell their patients their diagnosis, though some clinicians may accomplish this task better than others. Some clinicians will artfully explain the disease with compassion and sensitivity. If that is your experience, count your blessings. Others are sometimes not as fortunate.

A prudent caregiver will be proactive, visit the clinician, and discuss the details of how, when, where and why the diagnosis will be delivered. This is definitely a situation that will be accomplished better with appropriate planning. I recommend that this section be discussed with the clinician. However, caregivers should be sensitive to the clinician's professional feelings and emphasize that their primary concern is preventing the loved one from spiraling into severe depression.

Depending on the needs of your loved one, the common sense advice on these pages may be the most important in this entire book. As with any other advice, these are based solely on my experiences as a caregiver for Laura and not because I have had any medical training.

The primary caregiver should be present to provide support when the diagnosis is delivered. The presence of one additional/secondary caregiver or family member should be considered to provide extra support but no more than one.

Ensure the setting is private, quiet and interruption free. There should be no extraneous noise or distractions. If a desk or table is present in the room, it should be cleared of all items to minimize distractions. Naturally, cell phones should be not present or be silenced. This is an important medical conference and may be the most important one that the loved one will ever attend in his or her entire life.

The clinician should speak slowly, clearly, distinctly and direct his comments directly to the loved one receiving the diagnosis. Both should be seated, relaxed and on the same level. The doctor should maintain eye contract throughout the discussion only with the loved one, avoiding eye contact with the caregiver. The doctor should completely understand that the loved one receiving the diagnosis is the most important person in the world at this moment and deliver the diagnosis accordingly.

Only one message at a time should be provided by the clinician at a time who then pauses to give each message time to be clearly understood and processed. The clinician should pay attention to how the loved one is receiving the message and attempt to use empathy to learn their feelings. What is communicated back to the clinician by the loved one's use of words, gestures, facial grimaces, eye contact and other body language is important and should be sensitively received. When the loved one is speaking, neither the clinician nor the caregiver should interrupt unless help is requested to find the right word or finish a sentence. The clinician should consider having available a few water bottles to offer as a measure of both courtesy and compassion. Tissues should be readily available in the event tearfulness occurs.

This is a highly important personal matter. Literally, it is important life and death information so the clinician should maintain seriousness throughout the conference but maintain a relaxed composure and be in control. If the loved one expresses anxiety, the clinician should listen respectfully and then use diplomacy to defuse any extreme emotions.

The clinician should allow time for the loved one learning the diagnosis to absorb the information and to ask questions. If the loved one retreats into a shell or is shocked into silence resulting in having no questions, the clinician should advise what the most common questions other patients have and provide clear answers. The clinician should communicate a future game plan for the loved one and the caregiver to consider.

Once the clinician is clear that the loved one has learned and understood the diagnosis, the conference should be concluded. However, the loved one and the caregiver should be advised that they may continue to remain and use the private conference room as long as necessary.

The loved one may forget what the clinician said during the meeting, but will never forget how he or she felt when learning the diagnosis.

The minutes, hours, days, weeks, months, and years after and how to deal with them:

As time goes by, discussing dementia with your loved one is difficult. It may be best to allow your loved one to face the question however they personally choose. That being said, a useful recommendation is to allow your loved one to take the lead in their own dance. Another way of looking at this is to learn to let go of your reality and meet them where they are in the moment. That is, try to see the world through the eyes of your loved one who is living with dementia.

For a time, your loved one will dwell on the diagnosis. Think tender loving care – TLC – and spend as much time supporting your loved one as possible. Do activities together. Seek out pleasant movies, concerts, stage shows and local events. Visit relatives and friends. Exercise, pray, meditate and focus on the present. Naturally, it is best not to remind him or her of the diagnosis. However, in the event your loved one sometimes ask questions about what is wrong, it is important to handle these instances diplomatically and give as little information as possible. Over-explaining can lead to your loved one experiencing confusion and agitation. The dance goes on and your loved one is still leading. Follow his or her lead and if your toes get trampled, grin and bear it.

However, the loved one may press you with, "What is wrong with me?" At this point, only when directly asked, it is best to answer honestly about their condition. This technique is called reality orientation and is something that is usually only recommended during the mild stage or possibly early in the moderate stage. The key for the caregiver is to be able to adapt his or her approach on the fly by watching the loved one's behaviors and tone as the questions are being answered. If the caregiver notices agitation, combativeness, aggressiveness, long bouts of tearfulness or a determined fixation to ask repetitively about their diagnosis, then it is clearly time to use techniques other than reality orientation.

As the dementia disease progresses, the symptoms will intensify and your loved one may no longer dwell about their diagnosis. When this happens, allowing your loved one to lead in the dance means not reminding them of their condition. At this stage, your loved one may still sometimes ask questions about what is going on with them. It is important to handle these instances with a soft touch and give as little information as possible. Over-explaining can lead to confusion and agitation which may become a primary cause of anger. To handle confusion, repetitive questions, and the uncertainty about any other issues that arise, it is better to use alternate techniques such as distraction, redirecting to a different activity or reminiscing about positive experiences in their past.

Over time, your loved one will enter their comfort zone or emotional equilibrium. They will relax, slow down and eventually stop asking questions. Once your loved one enters this comfort zone, it is no longer necessary to address their diagnosis. Accept that your loved one is now leading in a slow dance. Each person and each journey are different, so you will likely go through a period of trial and error. Enjoy each day you have with your loved one as you enter their world and learn to dance with them.

Informing others about the loved one's diagnosis of dementia:

After receiving the diagnosis, who else should be told? Caregivers, family members and close friends are confronted with an enormously difficult decision when considering informing others about the loved one's diagnosis of dementia while in the mild stage. When informing others, the discussions are best accomplished one-on-one and not prolonged. No one wants to unnecessarily burden another person with excessive detail. Technical and medical questions are best left unanswered or referred to technical references, medical professionals or internet searches. Accepting the diagnosis in the minds of the caregiver, family and close friends is difficult, but it is natural for people to take some time to come to terms with the diagnosis. Some people will initially doubt the diagnosis, deny it or minimize it in their minds.

Choosing honesty and openness often helps some loved ones living with dementia immensely. The right to be open and honest and not insist on maintaining personal privacy is neither completely right nor completely wrong. Honesty and openness combine to support a valid psychological strategy and coping mechanism. The loved one living with dementia has the right to announce to the people in their world whom they love and respect that they have an incurable disease. Then this circle of important people in their life can support their efforts to combat it and to better prepare for the future. Everyone can hope and pray that the symptoms resolve or a cure is found before the disease becomes severe and it is too late. It is mentally much healthier to be optimistic than it is to be pessimistic. Hope springs eternal. Worldwide, there are hundreds of thousands of researchers working full time to find a cure for dementia diseases and for ways to slow its progression.

Since there is no cure ... and no effective measures to slow the progression ... some loved ones living with dementia choose the path of least resistance and not talk or think about it. It is a highly personal matter, extremely difficult to explain to others, emotionally charged and highly stressful to confront. For these and other reasons, dementia becomes the elephant in the room.

Countless people living with mental illness also live in secrecy. They refuse to disclose their illness to even close family members and friends. Many spouses of people with mental illness support this secrecy for fear of repercussion, spousal support and lack of a better alternative. However, others take the opposite approach and clearly inform many others. The middle ground is not always clear. There are no set rules of who should be told and when. Essentially, those who have a need to know and who will provide support should be told. By announcing the diagnosis to family, close friends, good neighbors, and members of your church and social groups, you and your loved one can receive support, understanding and assistance.

What Worked for Us That May Work for You

- There is a time for secrecy and denial. We chose this time carefully and well.
- We focused on enjoying each day we had together. There were many good days.
- We enjoyed visiting family, friends, neighbors, church groups, restaurants, grocery stores, clothing stores, consignment shops and décor specialty shops. Every day was a different adventure.

- We traveled extensively both to Europe and throughout the U.S. The adventure of self-guided travel was our passion.
- We found that saying little or nothing at all was the best way for us to approach each day from the dementia disease perspective. Once we knew Laura had dementia, we found that it was more important to focus on the journey in front of us than it was to discuss the disease.

Positive Affirmations

"Being deeply loved by someone gives you strength, while loving someone deeply gives you courage." – *Lao Tzu*

"One person caring about another represents life's greatest value." – *Jim Rohn*

End Note

[1]   Alzheimer's Dementia Journal, Early dementia diagnosis and the risk of suicide.
https://www.doi.org/10.1016/j.jalz.2009.04.1229
https://www.aanddjournal.net/article/S1552-5260(09)

CHAPTER 16

The Right to Personal Privacy

"You don't get to choose how you're going to die or when.
You can only decide how you're going to live."
– Joan Baez

Personal privacy is a funny thing. On one hand, everyone deserves that respect. But when you're dealing with dementia, sometimes the only way to offer that respect is to step over the line and into your loved one's space. Who knows better: The loved one actually living with dementia, you or someone else? Step into your loved one's shoes and think about personal privacy from their viewpoint.

I believe it is best to permit the loved one to deal with dementia however they personally choose. It is their life. I believe that how he or she wants to live it should be their personal prerogative.

The Difficult Decision

Many people who live with mental illness live in secrecy, refusing to disclose their illness to even close family members and friends. Some spouses of people with mental illness support this secrecy for fear of repercussion, for spousal support and for lack of a better choice.

Caregivers, family members and personal physicians are confronted with an enormously difficult decision when considering the formalization of a diagnosis of dementia, especially while the loved one is living with dementia in the mild and early moderate stages.

Since there is no cure and no effective measures to slow the progression, it is simply the path of least resistance to not talk about it and not think about it. It is a highly personal matter, extremely difficult to explain to others and highly stressful to confront.

For these and other reasons, dementia becomes the elephant in the room. Very few people with mild dementia and their caregivers are open about it. Both the loved one living with dementia and their caregiver(s) hope and pray that the symptoms resolve or a cure is found before the disease becomes severe and it is too late. It is mentally much healthier to be optimistic than it is to be pessimistic.

Our Future Financial Planning

Laura suspected she was living with dementia early in the disease. She had detailed knowledge of dementia because a close friend of ours had Alzheimer's disease dementia. Laura's mother lived with vascular disease dementia. It seemed as if the gene was inherited by some of her siblings. Her oldest brother lived with Parkinson's disease which became Parkinson's disease dementia at the end. We drove her other brother to a specialized center for brain scans which showed his advanced vascular disease. Her next older sister had Alzheimer's disease dementia and her oldest sister was a life-long special needs person who had many of the symptoms of dementia in her final years.

Another older sister had dementia at an advanced age. Although each of Laura's relatives lived a long drive from our home, we visited each one several times every year. After they showed symptoms of dementia, Laura was visibly shaken by each visit. However, she clearly felt a strong need to see them, talk to them and verify their care was adequate. Her sense of responsibility, obligation, love and duty to family was strong.

When dementia is suspected, but not yet formally confirmed by a diagnosis, long-term nursing care insurance can be considered.

When Laura was showing the early symptoms of dementia, I strongly suspected she was eventually going to face severe dementia due to her family history. Consequently, I spent considerable time searching the internet, making numerous telephone calls, sending out and answering many emails and eventually found an agency that would sell us long-term care insurance. Here's how I broke the news to Laura:

"Honey, I found an insurance agent that believes he can sell us a long-term care policy. It'll cover three years of care for either of us."

Laura replied, "Why would we want to spend money on that? Neither of us wants to go to a nursing home."

I countered, "Yes that's true, no one does, but all our friends have these policies and are happy they have them."

Laura said, "They can do whatever they choose. I don't want to waste money on something we'll never use."

I explained, "The agent thinks we qualify. He'll have to send a nurse to our home to verify we are OK."

Laura loudly and forcefully said, "When that nurse comes, I'm going to talk and act crazy. When I finish with that nurse, they won't sell us a nickel's worth of insurance, so you might as well forget that idea right now." Laura then added, "Remember, our business is our business. There is no sense in thinking otherwise. Keep that straight!"

I pushed back by saying, "It's not only for nursing home expenses, it's also for care at home in the event one of us is disabled and needs help. What if I have a stroke and become bedbound?"

"Nonsense," Laura added, "your mother took care of your dad for years after he was bedbound because of a stroke, so we will do the same. I will take care of you right here in this house and you will take care of me here, too. It happens all the time and that's what our all friends do, too."

Laura's mind was firm on this issue. Her desire to be cared for in our home and not in a nursing home was never in dispute. I brought it up a few additional times, but did not dent her armored resolve.

The expense of long-term care insurance must be carefully evaluated versus the availability of family members who can provide care at minimal cost. The loved one's assets may be sufficient to be self-insured or the loved one's assets may be minimal (already or almost impoverished) so that governmental social programs will pay for this type of care.

I reconciled myself to allocating our joint assets to pay for our needs as necessary and began financial planning accordingly. I converted our financial investments to very conservative choices. Since we started married life without any financial assets, the worst we could do was end our lives impoverished which would be a break-even for us.

Laura Exercised Her Right To Not Be Formally Diagnosed

It is clear that a person living with dementia has the right to know the diagnosis. Murkier is the reality that they also have the right to NOT know their diagnosis if that is their clear and informed preference. Laura understood she had the right to not be diagnosed, so she never was until the severe stage when it became a non-issue.

Sometimes saying little or nothing at all is the best way to approach each day from the diagnosis perspective. Once your loved one has been diagnosed with dementia, it is more important to focus on the journey in front of you both, than it is to discuss the diagnosis with them.

The right to not be formally diagnosed can be an extremely

effective strategy to avoid being caught up in a personal tornado of doubt, uncertainty, emotional turbulence and stressful discussions.

The symptoms could be caused by any one of numerous other disorders. Our personal care physician clearly understood this issue and began an attempt to rule out these conditions, one by one, through a comprehensive series of tests over a lengthy period.

The emotional toll of learning that he or she has a dementia diagnosis could be immense on a person. Some fall into severe depression and contemplate suicide when they learn they have a fatal disease for which there is no possibility of a cure.

Laura felt there was nothing anyone could do about it, so she took the necessary action to be not diagnosed with a dementia disease.

Laura Chose Personal Privacy

The maintenance of personal privacy is a strategy that many people choose in the mild stage. The loved one living with dementia has the absolute right to maintain personal privacy.

As you saw earlier in this chapter, Laura was highly familiar with dementia. My father also had dementia in his final year. My mother had mild cognitive impairment for her final years, but still lived independently. Many of our friends faced dementia at the ends of their lives. For us, it was nothing but a normal thing that most people faced.

When well-meaning friends would ask about her family's health issues, Laura suffered emotional pain. And rightfully so since Laura was action oriented. She had a bias for taking care of business which meant that she wanted to fix it. Make this disease pack up and leave town. However, there was nothing she could personally do to resolve their health issues. If there was, Laura would do it! She did not want to enter a spiral of self-pity and negativity by discussing the incurable illnesses of her loved family members. It hurt her to think about it.

Laura chose not to talk about it and not to think about it. I respected Laura's choice. She often privately said to me, "My business is my business!" And when I pushed back and said that her business affected me also, she countered with, "Our business is our business, and no one else's business! No one needs to know our business. Keep it that way!" Laura was strong-willed and assertive! It was easy to understand her personal wishes and preferences.

The use of the word "our" instead of "me" was clearly meant to convey that she and I were a unified team. Her expectations of my role were clear. We both suspected she had the beginning of dementia. But I was not to tell others. Laura was the clear leader on this matter and I was expected to support her 100 percent on this sensitive subject. Laura and I have always stood together facing life's problems encountered in our marriage. We were united on this issue also, rarely discussed it and both hoped for the best. It was her choice and she never failed to clearly communicate that.

Laura also used the analogy that we should never "air our dirty laundry in public." Laura chose to not disclose her illness because she did not want special attention. She didn't want people feeling sorry for her. Laura did not want to be entangled in discussions with well-meaning friends. She felt that talking about it would make her feel worse. I supported her decision and felt that it was a valid psychological coping strategy.

She firmly believed it would be counterproductive to announce that she suspected dementia had struck and then be engaged in conversations with worried friends. Also, since dementia brings about subtle, gradual and insidious changes which occur slowly over a period many years, the dementia was mostly invisible to others. Most friends accepted Laura's changes as normal aging. Laura and I followed the adage, "never complain, never explain. Your friends don't need it and your enemies don't care."

Life goes on. Laura knew she had dementia without hearing a diagnosis but since she was emotionally a very happy person, she was fortunately spared from severe depression.

Family members feel very protective of their loved one and often wish to spare them the trauma of dealing with a confirmation of a dementia diagnosis. Naturally, I would do anything to protect Laura and, fortunately, family and friends also did many things which also served to help and protect her.

Laura knew that once the diagnosis was made, family and friends were usually informed. Sometimes, when she was conversing with well-meaning people, they said the wrong thing and the blunder made her feel worse.

Laura feared the stigma of dementia. The complexity of openly announcing a diagnosis of dementia is compounded by the stigma attached to all mental illnesses by society including progressive neurological brain diseases. Laura felt that once people learned of it, they would shun both of us and our isolation would increase. There's much truth in that opinion. The Irish have a saying that goes like this:

> "When the specter of dementia enters your cottage, friends and family disappear like the morning dew!"

They often do! But social isolation did not occur to Laura. She had many friends and socialized with them whenever possible.

Other Challenges

Diagnostic uncertainty is a reality in some cases when certain specialized tests are not covered by medical insurance. Laura pre-empted specialized tests and exams by frequently making the comment that all doctors want is our money. When I pushed back and advised that we had excellent insurance that would pay for everything, Laura would then expound on the wasted time visiting doctor's offices and the aggravation of waiting for a long time for our turn. It was her way of justifying that specialists were NOT to be consulted. I understood this feeble rationale but also understood her strong desire to maintain personal privacy.

What Worked for Us That May Work for You

- Worldwide, there are hundreds of thousands of researchers working full time to find for a cure for dementia diseases and for ways to slow its progression. I hoped they would find a cure for Laura.

- We lived in the here and now. Today was our most important day. We focused on enjoying each day we had together. There were many good days. This hour was our most important hour. This minute was our most important minute. Tomorrow will take care of itself.
- Together, we enjoyed visiting family, friends, neighbors, church groups, restaurants, grocery stores, clothing stores and décor specialty shops. Every day was a different adventure. We probably had more quality time together during Laura's journey through dementia than we did during the preceding years.
- There is a time to exercise the right to personal privacy. We chose the present as this time.
- Much later, we found there was a time for a formal dementia diagnosis. We chose that time carefully and well.
- Much later, we found there is a time to communicate the reality of the diagnosis widely and openly ask for support from family, friends, neighbors and agencies. We chose this time judiciously.
- There is a time between these two extremes when very close family, very close friends, and medical specialists are clearly informed. We chose this time with precision.

Positive Affirmations

"Family is not an important thing. It's everything." – *Michael J. Fox, Actor*

"The simple act of caring is heroic." – *Edward Albert, Actor*

"Care is a state in which something does matter; it is the source of human tenderness." – *Rollo May, psychologist*

CHAPTER 17

The Right to Exercise Denial

"Always remember you are braver than you believe,
stronger than you seem, and smarter than you think."
– Christopher Robin

Is Denial a Negative Behavior?

Many people think of denial as a negative behavior. It is sometimes, but not always. If you have dementia, sometimes the best way to deal with it is to use your right to deny it affects you. You have that option. Exercising it is your choice. If you prefer, just ignore dementia and deny it affects you. Think about something else. There is actually no such thing as dementia if you don't think about it. You are as normal and healthy as everyone else.

Does this surprise you? It shouldn't. This choice is actually common in the mild stage. The loved one living with dementia has the absolute right to deny any problem exists. Actually, it is completely normal for most people in the mild stage to deny they may have a dreaded disease called dementia. Denial is a useful psychological defense or coping mechanism for both caregiver and loved one since dementia diseases cannot be slowed, improved or cured.

Much later in the progression, toward the end of the moderate stage and through the entire severe stage, denial is the only choice. In those stages, if you discuss the reality of the loved one's dementia disease, they will become despondent and suffer for a period of time. But, later, they will forget the discussion. So why be cruel and force them to think about the reality of their terminal illness? There is nothing to be gained. The medical term for this is anosognosia. It means a lack of awareness that a person has an impairment. The caregiver supporting the loved one's choice of denial may take comfort that it is only a phase. Other phases will follow as certain as night follows day.

Denial is a useful strategy used to reject something that your loved one wants to ignore or avoid because it is too difficult to face. It is difficult for the average caregiver to accept that their loved one chooses to refuse to recognize his or her impairment. Understandably, this can drive some caregivers to distraction. But your loved one has the absolute right to choose to deny any problem exists.

Many people fear dementia, and rightfully so. Can you imagine anything more fearful than being informed that you will progressively decline and lose your ability to remember those around you? That you will lose control of every aspect of your life? That you came into life drooling and pooping in your pants and that you will soon be leaving life drooling and pooping in your pants? What could be much scarier than facing that reality?

I am not a trained psychologist or psychiatrist, but I believe that this fear and the associated denial response is a wonderful psychological coping mechanism. A person simply does not have to think about it and therefore may feel that the problem does not have to be dealt with. It provides a measure of peace to an individual for a period of time.

The Clear Choice for Us: Denial and Secrecy vs. Honesty and Openness

Laura choose denial and secrecy. I supported her. Due to the force of her will (and my love for her), we stood together on this monumental problem. I thought back to our conversations on long-term care insurance and Laura's adamant opposition. Laura was totally negative on that concept. I believe it was part of her psychological denial strategy.

The concept of reality therapy is avoided if this choice is made. Reality therapy is hard, formidable, effortful and difficult. Denial is easy, simple, effortless and straightforward. There's a handy saying: "If you go looking for something long enough, you'll probably find it." Laura and I decided to not look for it. It is a smooth, downward path when denial is employed.

Laura did not want to lose the very important psychological benefit of denial and used this psychological crutch to the maximum. She was world-class on using denial to not focus on dementia and to direct her attention to other more enjoyable aspects of daily life. Laura never dwelled on her problems. She used her intelligence to do work-arounds. She was never shy about asking me for assistance.

What's Wrong with Denial

I am not advocating denial and secrecy for everyone. I am only explaining that it worked for us for a period of time and it may work similarly for some others. But for still others, the complete opposite may be the best approach.

Most experts will advise that denial as a coping strategy will eventually fail. I have no dispute with that position, but the most important consideration is your loved one's choice. If he or she chooses denial, thank the experts for their input and support the decision that is best for your loved one.

Denial has to be balanced with other important priorities. Completion of legal forms must go forward even though you and your loved one utilize denial. Simply explain that all seniors have to have these forms in order and it is a task that simply must be accomplished.

Reinforcing the reality that the caregiver is there for the loved one, will support them in every way and is dedicated to helping them is of paramount importance. Denial may work to help the loved one some, but the caregiver can work to help them much more.

Other health issues must be resolved and not ignored.

Denial may cause stress to the caregiver to the extreme that a heart attack, stroke or other serious health event could occur. This is a reality that must be faced. Denial may be too stressful for some caregivers. Sometimes denial causes major conflict within a family. Some family members may be strong advocates of reality therapy while the main caregiver is opposed to that strategy and supports denial.

What Worked for Us That May Work for You

- In numerous experimental studies, dementia diseases have been caused to occur in laboratory mice who are then later cured. I earnestly hoped that someday, some-how, these discoveries may be modified so they could work on Laura.
- I decided my job was not to convince Laura of the problem but to focus on what would keep her safe, happy, and healthy.
- We were united on this issue, rarely discussed it and hoped for the best.
- Was our decision right or wrong? We believed that, with personal decisions involving dementia, there are no absolutes. We believed that there was no moral dilemma involved in denying and concealing Laura's dementia. We believed that it was her personal choice and preference. Morally, we closed the case and ignored the complex ethical considerations.
- Was our decision common and does it happen often with people living with dementia? Or was it unique and happen seldom and rarely? We felt that with dementia there are no absolute decisions. There are no common issues or any perfect best practices to follow. Since no two persons living with dementia are the same, personal decisions are enormously complex.
- We lived in the here and now; today was our most impor-tant day. We focused on enjoying each day we had together.

There were many good days. This hour was our most important hour. This minute was our most important minute. Tomorrow will take care of itself.

- There was a time to exercise the right to secrecy and denial. There was a time to use the psychological crutch of denial. We chose the timing of each of these with great care.

- Much later, we found there was a time for openness and honesty. That was the time to communicate the reality of the Laura's illness widely and openly ask for support from family, friends, neighbors and agencies. We chose this time with care as well.

- There is a time between these two extremes when very close family, close friends and medical specialists are clearly informed.

- I kept a record of Laura's progression and furnished it in a private envelope at each of our routine six-month follow-up health appointments. Our primary medical doctor was kept informed so I felt my complicity and responsibility for the denial strategy was mitigated.

- Naturally, I felt guilty because I was unsure of the best approach. Consequently, I purchased and read numerous books on the subject of dementia, improving my knowledge and expertise considerably. I chose to educate myself on being a caregiver for a loved one living with dementia.

- The Internet has a wealth of information but it also has numerous blogs that only serve as venting platforms for caregiver frustration. Once I understood that some of the blogs were nothing but online pity parties, I avoided them. I found many were simply an exercise in "isn't it awful" and "my experience is worse than yours" by overwhelmed caregivers. I found they were nothing but depressive games (who has it worse, you or me?) that people were playing with each other. Sad, but true. I hope my book will help some of these individuals.

Positive Aspirations

"Family is the most important thing in the world." – *Princess Diana*

"I am not afraid of tomorrow, for I have seen yesterday and I love today." – *William Allen White*

"God grant me the courage not to give up what I think is right even though I think it is hopeless." – *Chester W Nimitz*

"Creativity requires the courage to let go of certainties." – *Erich Fromm*

CHAPTER 18

Advance Planning

"A good plan today is better than a perfect plan tomorrow."
– George S. Patton

It's important for all seniors to plan for the future and the plans be flexible enough to resolve unexpected issues. However, when a senior has dementia, it is vital that considerable planning be accomplished. Naturally, the senior must be legally competent to have the necessary legal capacity (the ability to understand the consequences) to participate, discuss alternatives, evaluate, arrive at informed decisions and to properly execute the decisions by signing various legal documents.

The downside of not planning can be severe.

When Laura was single, she had a successful career as an accounting clerk for a large corporation. Laura became friends with an older lady who worked there; they bonded and formed a mother/daughter-like relationship. After our marriage, Laura kept in contact with her and eventually became our daughter's godmother. Although we lived a long distance away, whenever we visited her city, we usually visited her home to socialize and I too became friends with her and her family. Eventually, we knew she was declining and showing signs of dementia.

Laura's friend now lived alone and had become isolated after her second husband, one son and daughter-in-law had died. The other son was seriously ill and lived in a distant city. Laura would call our friend periodically to chat but eventually could not reach her because the phone line had been disconnected. Also, Laura could not reach anyone who could give an update so she decided to visit her in person.

We traveled there and found our friend in a home that needed major exterior maintenance. The interior was filled with clutter and contained partially eaten spoiled food on the table and counter tops. It was a mess and totally unlike the previous visits when we found our friend's home well maintained and neat. The locks on the doors to her home were broken. A nearby neighbor saw our car there and came over to advise Laura that her friend's home was being visited by homeless men who routinely slept there at night.

We also found a sign declaring that the house was being foreclosed due to non-payment of property taxes. We knew that, early in the second marriage of our friend, the new husband convinced our friend to title the home in both their names. He also titled his business in both their names. We learned later that he and she took loans out to keep their business afloat with our friend as a co-signer on the loans initiated by her husband using their home as collateral. Then, several years later, the husband became ill, his business declined and he stopped paying taxes on their business. Unfortunately, he died from his illness before he could resolve the tax issue. What a complex mess!

Laura took charge. She made repeated calls to the local Social Service organization, but they were ineffective even after Laura became assertive and was transferred to the next higher supervisor. Eventually, she learned that the Social Service organization required a close blood relative to file a complaint before they could take action. This was not possible in this case. Laura also called the police but learned that law enforcement could not respond because no laws were being violated.

Laura made one final call and thankfully reached a different but knowledgeable lower-level person in the local Social Services organization. Laura told her story again, almost in tears at this point. The employee offered advice that was off the record and confidential. This person advised that Laura should simply call the emergency 911 number, report her friend as having a serious illness and request an ambulance take the woman to an emergency room for health reasons. Once at the hospital, laws would require that the medical establishment evaluate her and, if found incompetent, then give our friend proper care in a safe location. Laura made the call and our friend was transported, hospitalized, diagnosed and became the responsibility of the state. She was eventually relocated to a nursing home having an Alzheimer's wing. Laura also coordinated with the local police to nail the doors and windows shut to secure the home from trespassers.

The story does not end there. For the next eight years we visited our friend periodically at the nursing home where she was residing. I always complied with the nursing home requirement to sign the visitor log to document our visit. Sadly, during those eight years, only one other name besides my own was ever signed in the record book. It was a grandchild. Eventually, our friend became comatose and received nourishment and medications through a feeding tube for over a year. We discussed our friend's case with the nurses and they were willing to keep us informed. Our friend had bedsores, was obviously uncomfortable and in pain. She received prescribed medications for the infections and the pain but, to our untrained eyes, it seemed as if the treatment was ineffective. Laws of that state required life-sustaining medical treatment and prohibited ending a person's life if medical treatment was available to keep them alive.

Laura became an activist behind the scenes. She eventually located our friend's brother. No one had seen him in years but he'd recently moved back to the U.S. after retiring from a career in England. By that time, our friend's brother was her only living and responsible relative. Laura asked him to become involved and petition the state to perform a medical review of this case. To supplement his petition, Laura and I wrote a letter to document our personal knowledge. We never learned the outcome of the medical review or our letter's impact but soon our friend's soul was released from her body.

So, by our middle 40's, Laura and I were keenly aware of the downside of receiving extreme medical care in the terminal portion of the severe stage of dementia. Being comatose and in pain with no hope for recovery was not the future either of us wanted. We decided to avoid that possibility.

Laura and I both accomplished much of our necessary advance planning about this time, in our late 40s. We consulted an attorney, made wills, discussed burial alternatives and decided on how we would pay for our care. This was several decades prior to Laura entering the mild stage of dementia.

We even discussed the possibility of purchasing long-term care insurance, but discarded that planning option. Neither of us wanted nursing home care to be part of our futures. We decided to self-fund our future needs and promised each other care in our home as needed.

We finished our planning when Laura was in the mild stage of dementia in her 60's, but she clearly understood that the planning applied to both of us. We both agreed to all specifics regarding the powers of attorney and end-of-life wishes.

Planning for Possible Future Complexity

Seniors live in a complex world that can best be navigated through advance planning. The loved one living with early dementia, who assists their family to make his or her end of life preferences clearly known, is performing a great act of love. Completing the required legal paperwork can save the family from facing many needless issues, expenses and problems as well as save the loved one from needless suffering at the end of their life.

Does planning matter from a financial standpoint? The government is expected to do a vast amount to benefit all citizens, like:

- Regulate the economy, control the interest rate, minimize inflation, maximize employment, prevent recessions and balance the budget

- Become energy self-sufficient, solve global warming and eliminate water, air and ground pollution
- Make our highways, cities and other municipalities safer and improve health care
- Improve everyone's quality of life, end hate crimes, eliminate discrimination and racism and improve education
- Minimize terrorism, fight wars and help other countries

But, interestingly, the system of laws in federal and state governments do not subsidize long term care for loved ones living with dementia unless that person has very low income and asset levels. About three-quarters of what the federal government does is transfer payments. It collects revenue from income and payroll taxes and then sends checks either to households (for Social Security, pensions and welfare) or to health care providers (for Medicare and Medicaid).

Currently, it is my understanding that the federal government does not pay, and has no plans to pay [or even subsidize some of the cost for long-term health care] for a person living with dementia unless they are a very low income and asset level person.

Laura and I were retired seniors on a fixed income, but our income and asset levels were about mid-range for a married senior couple. We did not qualify for financial assistance for long-term health care although we needed this level of care.

Here are some questions I pondered as Laura took her mild stage journey. They are by no means to be interpreted as legal advice. Just some things to think about and some answers I came up with in my research:

- For married couples, does the caregiving spouse also have to also become impoverished (meet the low income and asset levels required by Medicaid law) prior to the loved one living with dementia being entitled to Medicaid? The answer becomes complex and depends on the state in which the married couple resides. In my state (NC), I understand all marital assets including jointly and individually owned financial assets, IRAs and 401Ks of both individuals must be spent down before Medicaid will make any payments for long term care.

- Should married couples with a high risk of one or the other developing dementia relocate to one of the states that does not require the spending down of all assets by both individuals? If so, what is the probability that that state will eventually change its laws to require a similar asset spend-down as my state requires? This is uncharted, unmapped murky territory.

- Should single seniors who fall in love with each other marry or should they simply informally commit to each other and form a domestic partnership? Simply stated, just live together and cohabitate. In my state, when an asset imbalance exists between the two individuals, it seems that forming a domestic partnership may financially be the better option from a long-term care cost perspective.

- Sometimes one or both of the single seniors have a special needs child or sibling they are committed to financially supporting. If they marry and are required to spend down their assets for the care of their spouse, then the special needs person's future expenses may not be met. Again, informally committing and forming a domestic partnership may be the better financial option.

- If they marry, does their state require both seniors to spend down their assets to the level of being impoverished in the event one becomes ill due to a dementia disease and requires long-term care? Naturally, the children and/or heirs of the spouse who has the most assets may not support marriage in this case. Forming a domestic partnership wins this round also.

- If two single seniors both have a secondary (to Medicare) health care benefit due to retirement from a previous career, would one lose that benefit if they married each other? Secondary health care policies are expensive so it is best to review and have a clear understanding of this issue prior to entering marriage. This situation may be somewhat rare but if it exists then a domestic partnership may be best.

- Naturally, I am not opposed to seniors marrying when they feel strong love and emotional commitment to each other. Also, the existence of a social stigma about living together, religious beliefs and personal values may prompt a high motivation to enter a traditional marriage. My research suggests that the couple also consider future detailed financial planning to ensure they are aware of any possible unintended consequences of marriage. Additionally, consulting an attorney skilled in advising seniors with financial issues may be helpful before tying the knot.

Can I Age in Place in My Home?

Aging in place is the most popular option for seniors including those loved ones who are living with dementia. Make plans accordingly, like:

- Downsize the home and its contents
- Clean out the clutter and emphasize priorities to reduce complexity
- Initiate part-time help and assistance as soon its needed

Mobility and other chronic issues may require an eventual decision for additional part-time care and, then, full-time, round-the-clock care may be needed. Become knowledgeable about these possible future realities. The vast majority of all long-term care is provided free by family members – that's plural on purpose – as we found that just one dedicated, full-time, 24/7/365 family caregiver is not doable.

Some families coordinate a rotational schedule among the various family members. I suggest you review the availability of home health aides in your community. There are numerous agencies that offer this service as well as many independent contractors who are equally or better qualified. Several part-time individuals may be feasible but your loved one may be better served by minimizing the amount of people who help them. Having different people caring for your loved one may cause confusion and increase his or her anxiety.

If family members working for free is not feasible, there are other alternatives. One is the expensive continuing care retirement communities (CCRCs) that offer different levels of service and charge accordingly. Another is remaining in one's home with full-time paid caregivers. Naturally, various professional agencies that specialize in this work can assume worker scheduling, coordination and the all personal care responsibility. Other families may choose to contract this work to a mother-daughter private contractor team who work out the availability schedule among themselves. Others may hire a private contractor where one person coordinates the schedules of several other private contractors to provide coverage on a 24/7 basis. But scheduling paid caregivers on a full-time basis is not feasible unless financial assets are significant.

Now is the time to discuss these thorny issues with everyone. Make certain your loved one's wishes are considered and his or her input is provided in answering these questions:

- How much will care cost and who will pay for it?
- Will the loved one have to spend down his or her financial resources? If so, how will this be achieved?
- Is there any equity in the home? Is there an insurance policy that can be accessed for funds?
- Are savings, investment resources or other benefits available? Is there a long-term care policy?

There may be other possible financial resources available if your loved one's financial resources have to be exhausted before State aid kicks in. For veterans and their spouses who become impoverished, VA benefits may be available. Eventually, Medicaid may be the only possible resource to cover the eventual cost of full-time skilled nursing home care.

As I mentioned above, I did a lot of research and found some answers to important legal questions you will face. Again, I'm not an attorney and not dispensing legal advice so please contact an attorney who has experience with these issues. These recommendations are **solely my opinion** as a former caregiver of a loved one living with dementia.

Do I need an attorney?

Yes, yes and yes! Always consider it necessary and prudent to utilize a professional attorney licensed to practice in your state to assist you in dealing with legal issues. Depending on the complexity of your situation and needs, a specialized geriatric or elder law attorney may be best or perhaps an attorney that deals in estates and wills. People with minimal financial resources may only need to consult with a general practitioner who has expertise with the Medicaid laws in your state. But people with considerable financial resources may need to consult with an attorney who routinely handles trusts and high asset estate issues.

Do I need a Will?

Yes, of course. I recommend that everyone have a Will. Laura and I had proper Wills prepared by an attorney. They were written in language that was clear, concise and reflected our wishes. Our situation and our Wills were simple and straightforward. We have what is known as a "sweetheart Will." We leave everything to each other. The survivor is the executor. After both of us dies, everything is then left 50-50 to our son, Michael, and our daughter, Sherri. They are co-executors.

Each individual has the right to make a decision on the need for a Will, but family members and/or heirs also have a responsibility to privately discuss this sensitive matter with the senior.

Do I need a Durable Financial Power of Attorney?

Yes! Naturally you will need to utilize an attorney. Laura and I had Durable Financial Power of Attorney documents drawn up years ago. At that time, we were each other's Durable Financial Power of Attorney. However, when Laura's symptoms of dementia became apparent, we changed my Durable Financial Power of Attorney to our son, Michael, who accepted this responsibility and our daughter, Sherri, who agreed to perform in this role if Michael is unable to serve.

I continued to be Laura's Durable Financial Power of Attorney, and we added the contingency that, if I was unable to serve, then Michael would become Laura's Durable Financial Power of Attorney with Sherri as the backup.

Do I need an Advance Directive?

Yes! But again, utilize an attorney. An Advance Directive is a set of instructions you state about the medical and/or mental health care you want if you ever lose the ability to make decisions for yourself. In North Carolina, for example, it is my understanding that there are three ways to make a formal Advance Directive. They are:

- A living will
- A Health Care Power of Attorney
- Advance instructions for mental health treatment

The increasingly popular Five Wishes Advance Directive form is available for most states via an online search. An attorney is not required to complete and implement this form.

What happens if you don't have an Advance Directive?

This can get very murky. I am not an attorney nor trained in the laws involving geriatric care, but it is my layman's understanding that:

- If you become unable to make decisions for yourself and have no Advance Directive, your primary medical provider or mental health provider will consult with someone close to you about your care.
- In the event of admission to a nursing facility, that facility will have the legal right to send you to the hospital if you become ill and require medical treatment above their level of care.
- In the event of admission to a hospital, that facility has the legal right and responsibility to perform all treatment necessary to sustain your life.
- In the event of an unresolvable dispute, legal action may be necessary.

Naturally, you and your loved one are encouraged to discuss your wishes with family and close friends and please consult with a lawyer to learn the specific rules in your state.

Do I need a Living Will?

Yes, you may need one, but you also need an attorney to prepare this document. To repeat, I am not trained as an attorney nor know much about the laws involving geriatric care. That said, I want to share my layman's understanding that a living will is a legal document that tells others that you want to die a natural death in the event certain circumstances occur such as follows:

- Become incurably sick with an irreversible condition that will result in your death within a short time.
- Become unconscious and your physician determines that it is highly unlikely you will ever regain consciousness.
- Have advanced dementia or a similar condition that results in very severe cognitive loss and it is highly unlikely that the condition can be reversed.

In a Living Will, it is my layman's understanding that you can direct your physician not to use certain life-prolonging treatments, such as a breathing machine (respirator or ventilator) and/or stop giving you food and water through a tube (artificial nutrition or hydration and IVs).

I think that it is logical to recommend that a Health Care Power of Attorney becomes effective only when your primary medical provider and one or more other physician(s) determine that you are unable to communicate your health care choices and determine that you met one or more of the conditions specified in the Health Care Power of Attorney.

Wow! These conditions and circumstances are extremely sensitive matters. Naturally, discussing a living will with your family is strongly encouraged.

Do I need a Health Care Power of Attorney?

Yes! But always consider the prudent action to utilize the services of an attorney to draft it. It is my layman's understanding that a Health Care Power of Attorney is a legal document in which you can:

- Name a person(s) as your health care agent(s) to make medical decisions for you if you become unable to decide for yourself.
- You can say what medical or mental health care treatments you want and do not want.
- You can choose and name the adult you trust to be your health care agent.

Again, I think it is logical to recommend that a Health Care Power of Attorney becomes effective only when your primary medical provider and one or more other physician (s) determine that you are not able to communicate your health care choices and determine that you met one or more of the conditions specified in the Health Care Power of Attorney.

Naturally, discussing a Health Care Power of Attorney with your family is strongly encouraged.

Do I need a Durable Health Care Power of Attorney?

Yes, definitely use an attorney for this document! In my research I have found there is a vast difference between a Health Care Power of Attorney and durable Health Care Power of Attorney. A Health Care Power of Attorney may be fairly short, simple and restricted to only a few matters. However, a Durable Health Care Power of Attorney is usually lengthy, complex and can widely cover many possible issues.

Laura and I had Durable Health Care Power of Attorney documents drawn that combines all concepts of an Advance Directive (a Living Will, a Durable Health Care Power of Attorney and Advance Instructions for Mental Health Treatment) all in one document. Three for the price of one!

Our advance directives were complex but written in language that is clear, concise and reflective of our wishes. They covered our end-of-life decisions. I was Laura's Durable Health Care Power of Attorney.

Durable Health Care Power of Attorney details to consider:

It is my layman's understanding that an attorney's detailed advice concerning a Durable Health Care Power of Attorney may include:

- In what circumstances, when, how, where and why will I direct that my health care providers and others involved in my care to provide, withhold or withdraw treatment?
- What if I have an incurable and irreversible condition that will result in my death within a relatively short time?
- What if I become unconscious and, to a reasonable degree of medical certainty, I will not regain consciousness?
- What if I undergo a marked lessening of my cognitive powers due to severe dementia, Alzheimer's disease, stroke or a sudden and permanent brain injury?

- What if my health care agent believes the likely risks and burdens of treatment will outweigh the benefits?
- What if my body has been seriously weakened by a progressive disease?
- When and in what circumstances will I direct that life-sustaining treatment be not given or be withdrawn?
- When and in what circumstances will I direct that I do not wish to be resuscitated (DNR)?
- What if pain medication fails to relieve all pain?
- What if I have major weight and muscle loss and my lack of appetite appears to herald cachexia (wasting syndrome).
- What if I have untreatable delirium?
- What if I am in a coma and unlikely to ever come out of it?
- What if I fail to recognize medical staff or friends?
- What if I stop swallowing solid food, or soft food or liquids?
- What if my swallowing reflex is completely lost?
- What if my sucking reflex is completely lost?
- When will I direct my health care agent to approve the withdrawal of all life-sustaining treatment?
- When will I direct my health care agent to ensure that I do not receive any fluid or food, whether by IV, tube feeding or other means?
- When will I direct my health care agent to ensure that I not be given Cardio Pulmonary Resuscitation (CPR)?
- When will I direct my health care agent to ensure that I not receive blood or platelet transfusions?
- When will I direct my health care agent to ensure that I not receive artificial nutrition?
- When will I direct my health care agent to ensure that I not receive dialysis?
- When will I direct my health care agent to ensure that I not receive surgery?
- When will I direct my health care agent to ensure that I not be placed on a ventilator or given intrusive diagnostic tests, including those requiring drawing my blood?

- When will I direct my health care agent to allow my wish to die naturally when I voluntarily stop eating and drinking (VSED)?
- How do I direct my health care agent to ensure that treatment for alleviation of pain or discomfort is to be provided at all times, even if it hastens my death or makes me lose consciousness?
- How do I direct my health care agent to ensure that I be kept fresh, clean and warm at all times?
- How do I ensure that my health care agent consults with a palliative care physician and that all recommended palliative procedures to ease my physical and emotional suffering be instituted?
- How do I direct my health care agent to ensure that I receive frequent position changes and meticulous oral, nasal and conjunctival hygiene? In this respect, insertion of a urinary catheter should be considered when approved by my physician.
- How do I direct my health care agent to ensure that I do not wish to be provided oxygen except as a palliative measure?
- How do I direct my health care agent to ensure that if I am in a hospital, to transfer me to a private room in a palliative care wing or equivalent?
- If I am not in a hospital or if transfer to the palliative care hospital wing or equivalent is not possible, how do I direct my health care agent to ensure my transfer to a private room in a skilled nursing facility that agrees to follow these instructions?
- If a skilled nursing facility is not possible, how do I direct my health care agent to ensure my transfer to the local hospice facility chosen by my agent?
- If none of the above is possible, how do I direct my health care agent to ensure my transfer to my home or to my health care agent's home, for private, skilled, palliative, nursing care augmented by hospice personnel?

Do I need a Revocable Living Trust?

Maybe. Again, think about being prudent and utilize an attorney. In this case, I believe it is mandatory due to the complexity of this type of trust. It is my layman's understanding that, depending on one's financial situation, this option may allow a person to keep control of all financial matters today and in the future and also provides an avenue to let the person of your choice take control in the future when certain circumstances are met, with a minimum of complexity.

I understand that a person has full control of their finances as long as they want and can make changes as often as desired. I believe what's included in the Revocable Living Trust document is exact language as to what situations may cause a person to be incapacitated and who will make the decision that you are incapacitated.

It seems like you can have your cake and eat it, too. In our case, Laura and I choose not set up a Revocable Living Trust. We learned that the initial attorney cost was high and then we would bear a periodic additional attorney cost for each update. We would have to put the title to our home and both of our automobiles in the trust as well as our IRAs, 401K, all bank accounts, all brokerage accounts, whole life insurance policies and all financial investments. Then, we understood that if we were to sell a car and/or buy a new one, close and/or open bank accounts, sell and/or purchase financial investments and the like, we would have to pay attorney fees to update the trust due to our financial asset changes. This seemed to us as too much cost and complexity for our relativity simple situation.

What Worked for Us That May Work for You

- We believed that, without a Durable Healthcare Power of Attorney, the person living with severe and end of life dementia makes it very difficult for their primary care physician to issue a Do Not Resuscitate (DNR) medical order.
- Here's what could happen: If and when Laura, having severe and end of life dementia, is signed into a hospital or nursing

facility, the medical staff there is required by law and their moral code to take all possible steps to extend her life. The typical action of a nursing facility for a person who is jeopardy of dying is to call 911 and transfer that person to the hospital. Once admitted to the hospital, extraordinary life-saving efforts would routinely be made. The hospital has full control. We were concerned about end of life pain and suffering issues. Essentially, we gained peace of mind by executing these Power of Attorney legal documents.

Positive Affirmations

"Faced with what is right, to leave it undone shows a lack of courage." – *Confucius*

"Planning is a process of choosing among those many options. If we do not choose to plan, then we choose to have others plan for us." – *Richard I. Winwood*

"Planning is bringing the future into the present so that you can do something about it now." – *Alan Lakein, Writer*

CHAPTER 19

Words Matter

"Of all the lessons I've learned through my years of caregiving the most important is to keep the love connection going. Just tell them that you love them again and again and again. You will never say it too much, ever."
– Joan Lunden

Laura was a natural talker and had strong interpersonal skills. Although her speaking and listening deficiencies began in the mild stage, she very effectively utilized her deep reservoir of life-long language and natural social skills. Consequently, it was almost impossible for others to recognize anything was wrong with Laura in normal social situations and conversations. Most friends and neighbors usually either did not recognize anything was amiss or simply attributed any speech issues to senior moments.

She also used her communication skills to effectively exercise her right to keep her dementia private. Also, her internal mental conversation and thought processes reinforced her emotional choice to deny having dementia. Naturally, close friends and family sometimes suspected something was wrong, but I consistently deflected their suspicions by advising that everything was fine with both Laura and me.

No one is born knowing how to properly communicate with their loved one living with dementia but they can learn. I did. It is difficult, but everyone can learn to use the unique communication skills needed to effectively communicate with a loved one living with dementia. They are vastly different from normal adult communication. Once fairly proficient in this area, I found that caregiving was much less stressful and it improved our relationship. My life became better and so did Laura's. Unfortunately, I learned them by trial and error. But I clearly acknowledge that knowing them earlier in the process would have been much better.

I eventually became a more effective communicator. As I became more proficient, our lives became more satisfying. Responding with a loving reaction usually disarmed, charmed, distracted and redirected Laura. Sometimes I was not able to successfully defuse an anxious situation. That was the worst-case scenario. The best case was that I sometimes inspired Laura to behave differently. Did Laura deserve my loving and kind responses? Of course. It was not Laura being difficult; it was the disease.

Some Things To Consider

Treat the loved one with love, respect, compassion and dignity:

I knew it was important to treat Laura with love, respect, compassion and dignity. I never talked down to her or spoke to her as if she were a child. When a third person was present, I would try to ignore the third person and focus on Laura. Later, I would excuse myself from the conversation to permit Laura and the third person to communicate one-on-one. When a third person was present and listening, I would only mention positive attributes of Laura. I would mention or acknowledge something in Laura's past that she did to lead a productive and useful life. I would reminisce and remind Laura of her accomplishments, especially if it was something that the third person could relate to. I tried my best to make Laura feel good about herself. I told her often that I loved her, because I did.

Sometimes Laura used malapropisms. They were not as powerful as Yogi-isms made famous by the great baseball player and coach, Yogi Berra. But they were clearly wrong words close in sound to the correct words. I usually jumped in the conversation and reinforced what Laura was saying, but I would use the correct word hoping that no one would ridicule her for mispronouncing the word. I was usually successful in maintaining Laura's dignity, as we both knew enough about it to continue the discussion if anyone was interested and I would downplay the mispronunciation.

Never argue when criticized:

I knew to never argue when Laura was personally critical of me. It never did any good and usually made things worse. Like most people living with dementia, Laura suffered personality changes and was prone to become irritable and easily agitated. Getting into an argument with her definitely heightened her agitation. I learned to thank Laura for her input and quickly admit my shortcomings. Naturally, I promised to correct my behavior in the future. After defusing the situation, I employed the wonderful tool of distraction and changed the subject and sometimes the environment. We might move together to a different room, take a drive or walk together. Here was my typical response to Laura's criticism: "Honey, I'm flawed. I make mistakes. I'm sorry. Thank you for sharing that with me. I appreciate you! I love you. Thank you for loving me. Oh, we are out of milk. Are you ready to go for a drive to the store?"

Control the communication and accent the positive:

I found that it was vital to keep my body language, facial expression, tone of voice, volume of my voice and physical proximity positive and pleasant. I did not confront Laura or get in her face no matter what circumstances or behavior occurred. I used gentle physical touch to connect and convey my feelings of affection when conversing to ensure Laura had my complete attention.

Set a positive mood for interaction:

I soon recognized that my attitude and body language communicated my feelings and thoughts stronger than my words. I focused on setting a positive mood by speaking to Laura in a pleasant and respectful manner. I used facial expressions, tone of voice and physical touch to help convey my message and show my feelings of affection. I learned that slow, cheerful, calming and reassuring speech was best.

Limit distractions and gain attention:

I learned to turn off the television, radio or music system when conversing. If it was distracting to Laura, I dealt with it. I found that a quiet place without distractions made it much easier to have a conversation. Laura was right-handed, so her dominant side was her right side. I eventually understood it was best to approach Laura slowly on her right side, then get down to her eye level or below her eye level. If she was seated, I would sit down next to her on the couch or pull over a chair close to her. I would always address her as "Laura" or "Honey" or both when I initiated a conversation. This seemed to ensure I had her attention and often said: "Laura, your husband Tom wants to have a chat with you." It is important to understand that a loved one's own name is something they will never forget and always love to hear.

Communicate with body language:

Body language facilitates two-way communication. I learned to maintain eye contact with Laura when conversing and to smile. I used gentle touches to her hand, forearm or upper arm to improve our physical connection at that moment. I found these non-verbal physical body language cues added value and meaning to the communication.

Sometimes, when I could not understand the point of what Laura was saying, I would ask her to point or gesture to augment her speech. I watched her eyes to see what they were viewing and used that information also to gain better understanding.

Remember, the person living with dementia can read your body language. If you steeple your hands as in prayer, they may suspect you feel superior to them. If your arms are crossed in front of your chest, they might feel you are rejecting them and do not want to be there. If you are rubbing your face, they may know you are feeling uneasy and unsure of yourself. If you are making faces, they know exactly how you are feeling. Laura maintained expertise in reading body language.

So, I had to learn Laura's body language. When she would not make eye contact with me or say anything to me, I was clearly being stonewalled. I found it was best to walk away for a few minutes, do some deep breathing, collect my wits, then return and retry to gain her confidence. I would approach her using my "guilty person" approach and offer a general apology since I usually didn't know what I had done to offend her. Then, I would change the subject to some pleasant topic.

Laura was always fastidious about personal appearance, breath smell and body odor. I always kept myself clean shaven, freshly showered, hair combed, teeth brushed and gums flossed. Naturally, I used mouthwash, underarm deodorant and applied after shave (but not too much).

I tried to keep my voice at a normal conversational speed, volume and tone: Not too slow, not too fast, not too low, not too loud, not too hard and not too soft. Sometimes, I found that if I spoke using a low, deep-pitched voice, that seemed to relax her when she seemed agitated.

Keep the conversation short, clear and simple:
I found that simple was best and used basic words, phrases and short sentences. I found that speaking slowly and clearly enunciating all words in a moderate and reassuring tone was effective. When it was clear that Laura did not understand the conversation, I repeated what I was saying by using different or better words to convey my meaning. I learned that being specific and using the exact names of people and places instead of general pronouns (thereby

avoiding he, she, they) was more effective but took more effort on my part. Naturally, I avoided using abbreviations and slang.

Keep questions simple:

When I asked Laura a question and she didn't understand the first time, I used simpler wording to repeat my question. If she still didn't understand, I would wait a few minutes and rephrase the question using basic common sense. I would repeat Laura's name, try to ensure both of us were relaxed, continued eye contact, kept that smile on my face and simply rephrased the question again. When I could not get my message across, I shifted to asking questions that only required yes or no answers.

A picture is worth a thousand words:

I soon recognized the value of giving choices and offering visual cues such as, "Do you want this glass of milk or this orange juice with your breakfast?" While helping her dress in the morning, I would go to the closet and pull out two pairs of slacks, saying: "Do you want to wear this pair of grey slacks or these navy-blue slacks today?" And, at breakfast, I would put her medications in front of her and say, "Here are your morning vitamin pills. Do you want to take them now or later?" This type of communication clarified the meaning of what was being communicated. Naturally, I avoided asking general or open-ended questions.

Be patient and listen with your ears, eyes and mind:

Since Laura's processing speed was slower, I learned to slow my speech to give her time to think about what she wanted to say. We both learned that a moment of silence is golden. When Laura was struggling to find the correct word or use correct pronunciation, I would wait for a moment and, if I felt it was appropriate, I would offer one that I thought she meant. This was done with empathy and never any criticism. Sometimes, I would rephrase what she was trying to say in my own words. I learned to closely watch Laura's body language and listen to the tone of her voice to learn the meaning of what she was trying to communicate and how she felt about it. I found that using patience and slowing down the conversation resulted in fairly effective and clear communication. If she was having trouble getting her point across, I would reassure her it was okay to sometimes have difficulty communicating. Occasionally, Laura lost her train of thought. I would calmly remind Laura of the subject she was just talking about. If she got back on track, that was fine and, if not, that was okay too. We would just go on to a different subject.

Listening with empathy:

I learned to listen with empathy as building trust as well as reducing anxiety and agitation is much more important than the actual words being spoken. I would try to focus and concentrate on Laura's feelings and needs. Often, the emotion behind what she was saying was much more important than the actual words she was using. Naturally, Laura had a need for recognition, self-worth, and identity. I did my best to be non-threatening and factual in everything I said.

Mirror back agitation, then distract, then redirect:

When Laura became frustrated, and expressed agitation or anger, I learned to accept the communication and mirror it back to her to ensure she understood I received her message. I would say, "I know you are upset about _____ and I understand your concern. I agree that it is awful. I am sorry you feel bad about _____. I feel bad about _____ too. Thank you for telling me about that."

I made a priority to learn what and how Laura was feeling before going forward with the standard tools of distraction and redirection.

Laura wanted to vent from time to time so I let her. As she expressed negative or difficult feelings, I would acknowledge them and that always seemed to help. Once I learned her feelings and felt Laura had vented enough, I then used distraction and redirection saying something like, "Oh, I wanted to let you know about what your grandson did last week at school. Sherri said he gave an oral report to this class and the teacher gave him an A. He is an excellent speaker, well-liked by his classmates and not shy at all." Or something like, "Hey, I just remembered that we need to go for a ride to the store and pick up something for our lunch. Can I help you get your coat on?"

Respond to negatives with positives:

I learned to respond to uncertainty, confusion, anxiety, falsehoods and other negativity with positive communications. When Laura was having a bad day, I found that making extra effort to be supportive, affectionate and reassuring really helped. Her confusion and communication about events that may have never occurred was difficult to understand, but I learned to focus on the feelings that Laura was communicating, not the facts. I discovered that any negative feelings being communicated by Laura were completely real to her and were best handled with me offering verbal and physical expressions of love, comfort, affection, support and reassurance. I eventually learned to eliminate any negatively from my remarks and never told her she was wrong.

I found that touching her hand, lower arm or upper arm usually helped communicate our connection. When she was very upset, I learned to hold Laura's hand, give her a hug and offer positive feedback. This seemed to help calm her down and improve her spirit. The phrase, "Let's do this instead," was invaluable.

Remembering the past:

Laura's memory of the past brought her much comfort during her mild stage. The past was the good old days. I hit upon asking her questions about her school days, her parents, her brothers and sisters, her friends, her early career, her choir group performances, our early marriage days when our children were small, her Shetland Sheepdog Scottie and the various sales positions she excelled in during our married life. Talking about the distant past brought back relaxing and enjoyable memories of her life. Laura had excellent recall of what happened a long time ago. Naturally, I learned to avoid asking questions that relied on short term memory such as asking her to comment on what she ate for breakfast or lunch.

Use humor:

I am not a joker and can't tell a good joke no matter how I try. But I do have an everyday wry sense of humor, especially when the joke is on me. I do recognize humor in everyday happenings both to me and in the world in general. I did my best to use humor every day but never at Laura's expense as that would have been cruel. Laura retained her social skills and was usually delighted to laugh along with me at many of life's humorous situations.

Repetitive speech issues:

Laura would often repeat a word, statement or question or activity over and over. This type of behavior was clearly harmless for her but it sometimes was annoying to our grandchildren. I did my best to defuse their stress when their grandmother made repeated comments or questions. I tried to answer each comment or question using a different phrase. I knew that repetitive speech is sometimes triggered by anxiety, boredom or some unknown fear or an environmental issue so I usually tried to determine the underlying cause.

What Worked for Us That May Work for You

- I never disagreed: I simply agreed and repeated what was said to convey that I understood. I didn't say, "You can't do that." Instead I said, "Let's do this instead."
- I never questioned: I listened and advised Laura that I loved her and was there to help her.
- I never lied: But I did sometimes use therapeutic fibs which were roundabout truth avoidance tactics.

- I never argued: I listened, agreed, and expressed sympathy if appropriate.
- I never contradicted or corrected: I listened and offered a comment that I understood sometimes repeating what Laura stated in my own words.
- I never shamed or condescended: I encouraged or praised desirable behavior. I distracted if appropriate.
- I never commanded nor demanded: I asked for and personally modeled the desirable behavior.
- I never expressed irritation: I remained calm and modeled patience.
- I avoided complexity: I kept everything simple.
- I never said: "Remember." I reminisced about experiences I thought were familiar.
- I never said: "I told you." I repeated and regrouped.
- I never said: "You can't." I found out what Laura could do and encouraged her in that direction.
- I never forced behavior: I reinforced the desirable behavior.

I used these golden phrases:

- "Are you hungry or thirsty?"
- "Are you comfortable or uncomfortable?"
- "Do you need help? What can I do to help you?"
- "Do you hurt? Where does it hurt?"
- "Are you tired? Do you want to rest?"
- "Do you want to sit or lie down? Let's both lie down and rest."
- "Are you too hot or too cold?"
- "Are you sad?"
- "Did someone hurt your feelings?"
- "I love you. How can I help you?"
- "Do you feel safe? I will keep you safe."

To communicate effectively, I would:

- Approach Laura slowly and sit closely by her on her dominant right side.
- Take and hold Laura's hand for a moment to relax her.
- Kiss Laura on the cheek to punctuate my greeting.
- Look Laura in the eye, soften my face by smiling:
- ...and softly say "I love you," "I will always take care of you," "I will always love you," "I will always keep you safe."

I found that I could not say these words often enough, but Laura would sometimes say to me, "I already know that," meaning I have repeated myself and I am wasting her time so I should quit repeating these words. But Laura's body language said something else. These words always generated a relaxed, soft smile on Laura's face. She liked hearing them. Who wouldn't? So, I said them often.

Positive Affirmations

"If you want others to be happy, practice compassion. If you want to be happy, compassion." – *The Dalai Lama*

CHAPTER 20

TLC Action Plan
Going Forward

"Live with intention. Walk to the edge. Listen hard. Practice wellness. Play with abandon. Laugh. Choose with no regret. Do what you love. Live as if this is all there is."
– Mary Anne Roadacher-Hershey

How to Take Care of You

I want to start this chapter with some important items to consider.

- Who is now and who will continue to be the much more difficult person to care for: You the caregiver? Your loved one living with dementia? Knowing what to expect will make it much easier for the caregiver to properly plan ahead. There will be problems faced and solutions found. They will all come within a caregiver's capability if he or she plans and prioritizes for them.

- Who is now and who will continue to be the person who is much more important in this caregiving situation: You the caregiver or your loved one living with dementia?

- Who is now and who will continue to be the person who has the most physical, spiritual, emotional and financial stress: You the caregiver or your loved one living with dementia?

The answers to these questions are not obvious. The typical care-giver has tremendous love and sympathy for the loved one living with dementia. I know I did. The caregiver knows the loved one can no longer enjoy life to the maximum and will most likely endure personal suffering in the future. Should the caregiver immerse him-self or herself in guilt over this certain eventuality. No! The future quality of life for the loved one is strongly dependent on the care-giver's health and well-being. The typical caregiver will be perfectly capable of properly caring for the loved one but often will not prop-erly care for themselves. I know I didn't.

Surveys show that about half of all caregivers describe their health as excellent or very good, while about half say their health is good, fair or poor. What is health? In these surveys, it is the caregivers' percep-tion of their personal physical, mental, spiritual and emotional health. However, as the caregiving burden increases to 24 hours/day and 7 days/week, caregivers often report their health deteriorates. The real-ity is that the average caregiver's health deterioration often increases over 20 percent. It is even higher for those caring for a spouse. Over 34 percent caring for a spouse report that caregiving has made their health worse. Those who feel they had no choice in taking on their caregiving responsibilities report 32 percent worse physical health. Caregivers of a loved one living with Alzheimer's or dementia also re-port over 32 percent health deterioration. Similar higher numbers are reported for those who care for someone for over a year or who have a higher-hour burden requiring 24 hours/day and 7days/week care-giving. Unfortunately, at least a third of caregivers of a spouse living with dementia will suffer worse personal health. [1, 2, 3]

Caregivers usually run a gauntlet of emotions. They may range from fear to courage, from joy to sorrow, from anger to happiness and from guilt to acceptance, compassion and understanding. Accept that taking care of yourself and protecting your normal hu-man emotions from depression is a high priority.

It's easy to say, "Put on your oxygen mask first," as if you were on a plane with a child, the cabin lost pressure and the oxygen masks dropped from their overhead storage. But in caregiving reality, it's not a one-time, well-recognized situation. It's a day-to-day, often stressful, usually demanding, decision-making lifestyle that can wear out some caregivers. If you are in the top two out of three who thrives on being a caregiver, skip the rest of this chapter. But if perhaps you are not the superman or superwoman type, read on carefully.

You'll be eaten alive by worry and stress unless you start and maintain adequate self-care. It's natural to focus on the loved one living with dementia but the reality is that the physical toll on caregivers over time is huge. Prioritize and schedule your own routine healthcare appointments for the next 12 months now and write them on your calendar in ink.

You are in a marathon, not a dash or sprint. It's natural to focus only on the person with dementia when symptoms are new. But it is counterproductive to ignore your life and needs for months or years. Don't put your life on hold.

Repetitive, annoying, aggravating, and/or rude comments aren't being said by your loved one on purpose. The dementia causes them. The less you and your loved one butt heads over things that can't be changed or controlled, the more you can learn how to work with the real adversary, the diseased brain. Learn the why behind common symptoms of dementia to help you redirect or avoid them.

Don't be too quick to give up your personal exercise routines, outings with friends, hobbies and other sources of stress reduction. Avoid rationalizing that you'll get back to them when the current crisis is over. The reality is that you will face a series of ever-changing crises in the future. You'll naturally require a few constant sources of personal enjoyment, support and strength.

Don't keep dementia a total secret from the world even if your loved one chooses personal secrecy as a psychological crutch. Confide in at least one person to whom you can freely consult or vent as needed. Vent online, too, but don't get caught up in the games some depressed and overwhelmed caregivers play on these on-line sites. I call them the "Isn't it awful!" and "My problems are worse than yours!" games. If you weren't depressed before you indulge in some of these internet pity sessions, you may be afterwards. If so, avoid the dementia venting blogs.

Exercise early in the day before time runs away from you. Good home-based choices include walking in the home and up and down stairs, floor exercises to stretch and strengthen, using exercise bands, lifting light hand weights, performing yoga and tai chi, using exercise machines and following instructor-led exercise DVDs.

Instead of attempting to change your whole diet, start with smarter snacking. Use the perimeter of grocery stores to purchase fresh or dried fruits, nuts, fresh vegetables, healthy dairy products, whole grain breads, popcorn, green tea and flavored waters.

How to Build Your Family/Friends/Hired Help Support System Network

You'll need more help as time goes by, not less. Even if you currently feel under control in your current TLC care plan, eventually your loved one's abilities to perform everyday tasks will deteriorate and you will be faced with ever increasing responsibilities. No single individual can manage dementia care for a loved one all the way through, all alone. Start now, even if you start slowly, getting help from others.

Your support network is an important part of being a caregiver. Start a master list of everyone who volunteers to help you or may be of help. People who drive, gardeners, errand runners, socializers, visitors, sitters and handy men are just some that come to mind. When you need help, turn to the list.

Call the various local Social Service Agencies, especially those who specialize on Aging to learn what resources are available in your community for caregivers of loved ones living with dementia. You may need them later so do it now to find possible reinforcements for your care plan.

If employed, inform your employer about what's going on. Some companies offer eldercare or other work-life benefits, flextime or dementia-specific educational resources. From what I understand, legally, caregivers are considered the same at work as a working parent.

Even if you're not a highly social person consider joining a support group for dementia caregivers. You'll learn strategies for communicating better, meet people who can relate, learn how you can find help, meet highly valuable contacts and much more.

You, not your loved one living with dementia, will have to change. Your emotional relationship with the loved one you care for will change despite all your love and help. As time goes by, everyone with dementia becomes more dependent. Old balances of power and home responsibilities will change dramatically. You'll always have great love for your loved one, but the emotional interactions will never be the same. Gradually, spousal love between two married people will change from love to friendship. Parent-child relationships will change as the child caregiver becomes the parent and the parent being cared for becomes the child.

Let yourself grieve a little. Your life has changed and will continue to change. It is beyond your control. Grief is normal and that is what you're experiencing even during the mild stage of dementia. You are gradually losing your loved one. It's extremely hard to see them slowly deteriorate, but you have no choice.

Embrace the good days, the good hours and good moments as they occur. Dementia doesn't instantly erase the fun, love, laughter and companionship in your life. Live in the moment as best you can. Find new ways to enjoy life. Force your mind to not dwell on unpleasant daily occurrences or disrupted future travel plans. Plan for future enjoyable experiences.

How to Take Care of Both of You

As an Alzheimer's advocate, I look for information on the Internet that is fascinating. I have summarized what I believe is the most important information into ten steps. I believe these steps may moderate the negative aspects of dementia. The same steps may also possibly slow the progression of dementia. I highly recommend that both the caregiver and the loved one living with dementia follow as many of these steps each day as possible.

When did I learn about the most important sources of information available on the Internet? I have reviewed this subject for over ten years. Dementia ran in Laura's family and I expected that she would eventually experience this disease. Since dementia is strongly correlated with aging, I believe that the majority of seniors who live a long life will eventually experience some form of dementia.

I tried many online recommendations to help Laura but none had much impact. Eventually, I suspected that most were bogus especially if the recommendations were accompanied with a sales pitch to purchase a product. Others were well-meaning attempts by individuals to simply offer possible steps or alternatives that might help. I found that most too-good-to-be-true Internet recommendations were debunked eventually by reputable researchers who diplomatically advise that their studies showed no benefit resulted from use of that product, step or alternative.

Many factors contribute to a caregiver's health and to the health of a loved one living with dementia. Often, the loved one exhibits challenging behavior. Following these steps may improve the health of both and serve to minimize and alleviate the loved one's challenging behaviors. You will find many similarities by carefully comparing these steps to the recommended steps in published information to minimize and possibly reverse cardiovascular disease. This is because improving or maximizing blood flow includes more blood flow to the brain. These steps may also serve to minimize harmful inflammation throughout the cardiovascular system including the brain. [4]

The Alzheimer's Association International Conference (AAIC) is the world's largest gathering of Alzheimer's disease (AD) and dementia researchers, physicians and health care professionals. The AAIC provides attendees with the opportunity to learn the latest in dementia research, findings and studies. It allows the participants to network with leaders in the field from around the world. I made a concerted effort to access and review the online information available from these meetings and to summarize what I believe is of value to the caregiver and to the loved one living with dementia.

I have reviewed the AAIC abstracts, reports and press releases going back over the last two decades. They are listed in the end notes to this chapter. If interested, caregivers may access them through an internet search of "AAIC ____ (year)." I used this information to develop a ten-item summary of steps to take better care for both the loved one and the caregiver. These steps should be considered by all seniors as a high priority. The difficulty is that they require personal commitment and discipline. Some of the experts at the AAIC meetings have stated that if the beneficial aspects of these steps could be put in a pill, it would be the most popular pill in the world. [5]

Here are my Top 10:

1. Follow a healthy diet. Choose either a plant-based diet or a vegan-type diet. If plant based is too difficult, then try the Mediterranean diet or the MIND (a hybrid of Mediterranean and low glycemic regimens) diet. All of these restrict fats to a moderate intake of healthy extra virgin olive oil and a very low intake of sugar. Body fat recommendations are usually easily achieved by anyone following a healthy diet.

2. Maintain blood pressure in normal limits. Include restricting sodium to not more than 2/3 of the recommended daily adult amount. This is difficult unless a person primarily buys fresh produce, uses herbs to season, and cooks at home. One restaurant entree will usually exceed this guideline, as do grocery store packaged and canned foods.

3. Enjoy positive socialization daily. The more you socialize, the better.

4. Sleep 7 to 9 hours per night. Emphasize maximum REM (dreaming) sleep. Be aware that more than one glass of wine for a woman or two glasses of wine for a man in the evening

hours will disrupt REM sleep. If any senior exceeds that amount or snores during sleep that person should consider a CPAP machine.

5. Relaxation, meditation, mindfulness and private spiritual prayer each day is important. Avoid stress whenever possible and live within your financial means.

6. Enjoy physical exercise every day. If possible, walk the recommended 10,000 steps per day, and do some stretching or yoga exercises and some strength training.

7. Remain in a happy, committed, loving relationship including a high degree of communication along with enjoyable mental, empathetic and physical intimacy.

8. Mental exercise is vital. Experience and master cognitive challenges: Become highly proficient in board games you enjoy, learn a new musical instrument, foreign language, take an interesting academic or adult learning course in a subject outside your normal area of expertise or read books outside your favorite genre.

9. Strive to follow all well-known and recommended physical, mental, emotional and dental health care preventive measures. Alcohol consumption should be moderate. Discontinue use of tobacco products as they have a wide spectrum of known negative health outcomes. Ban all illegal drugs from your life.

10. Take all prescribed medications and personal medical physician recommended non-prescription supplements.

How to Take Care of Your Loved One

First, adopt empathetic listening methods when conversing with your loved one. Empathetic listening is a general-purpose term with varied meanings. With respect to human emotions, it recognizes and accepts another person's thoughts, feelings, sensations and behaviors. In psychology, it expresses understanding and acceptance of another person's internal experience. It builds on positive emotions and thoughts. To listen empathetically does not mean you agree or approve. It means you are trying your best to understand what they are saying. It has tremendous value as it serves to build relationships and help ease upset feelings.

Laura lived with dementia and I remember how the disease progressed over the years. If I had known of the empathetic listening method early in my care for her, the knowledge and use of this method would have improved the quality of life for both of us. Empathetic listening is not the normal way that people are motivated. It lacks goal orientated direction and purpose. Everyone can become an empathetic listener, but it takes conscious effort, discipline and practice.

Caregivers eventually learn that they can't swim upstream against the swift, strong current of dementia or swim against its incoming rising tide. They learn that they must enter the water and swim with the current and tide. The caregiver must go with the flow! The most seaworthy vessel riding this flow is called empathetic listening.

A woman living with dementia must be treated as the most important Crown Princess of the kingdom. She is heir to the throne and will be the Queen someday. A man living with dementia must be treated as the most important Crown Prince of the kingdom. He is heir to the throne and will be the King someday. You treat royalty with respect. The royal person is unique and worthwhile. We accept the royal person as they are and do not attempt to change them. If they insist (and they may often will) on being spoiled, then spoil them! You never lie to royalty or anyone who is living with dementia. You listen to their words and if you disagree, you respond diplomatically and indirectly to whatever concept they are stating, or point they are making.

I believe the empathetic listening method discourages direct therapeutic fibbing but accomplishes the same result by making creative responses that provide input by using indirect speech. I think of this as round-about truth avoidance. It could also be called enhanced or indirect therapeutic fibbing. Does this sound confusing? It is confusing because it is counter-intuitive to our normal instincts of being efficient and direct in our speech.

Second, enter the loved one's world. Because loved ones living with dementia have serious cognitive impairments that cause difficulty communicating, it's challenging for caregivers to understand what they're trying to say. Here's how I believe you can manage conversations with your loved one living with dementia: Understand their world.

A loved one with dementia is living in a different reality from the caregiver. That reality can be scary and confusing. If our loved one keeps asking to see their deceased spouse, parent or sibling, they really do believe that person is alive. If no one is being hurt, it's okay to play along with their beliefs. Their mind has been taken over by a devastating disease and it has a profound effect on how they experience and understand the world. It's difficult for a mentally sound person to really understand what it's like to live with dementia.

What do you say to the loved one who asks to see a diseased relative? Think first and then say something like, "I know you love him (or her) very much. I haven't seen him (or her) for a long time. Maybe the next time we go on a trip, we can try to visit him (or her). Let me get you a glass of water. We are supposed to drink eight glasses of water every day."

Third, treat the loved one with respect and dignity. Don't talk down to your loved one living with dementia or talk to other people about them as if they weren't there. Communication and social skills gradually deteriorate. A loved one living with dementia sometimes may have trouble finding the right word. Very often they are aware that something is amiss, but they may not be sure what's wrong. They naturally avoid situations where they feel put on the spot or vulnerable to embarrassing mistakes such as social outings, time with friends, mentally challenging situations and sometimes even telephone conversations. While everyone occasionally forgets words or names during conversations, this problem occurs with increasing frequency in people with mild dementia. They may substitute or make up words that sound like or mean something like the forgotten word. They sometimes even avoid talking to keep from making mistakes and may sometimes appear subdued or withdrawn.

Fourth, use patience and compassion. Be generous with your patience and compassion. They are essential for communicating with your loved one who is often confused and sometimes frightened. Being caring, calm and positive can make a big difference for them. Gloss over mistakes. Assure the loved one you're there to provide ongoing love, help and support. Loved ones with mild dementia may experience memory loss, lapses of judgment and subtle changes in personality. They often have decreased attention span and less motivation to complete tasks. In addition, they may resist change and new challenges and get lost even in familiar places. The loved one may ask repetitive questions or hoard things of no value. When frustrated or tired, they may become uncharacteristically angry. Erase phrases like, "Try harder" or "You're not concentrating enough." The loved one with dementia is doing the best he or she can. Berating or cajoling only adds frustration and can lead to more mistakes.

Memory lapses are typically the first sign of early mild stage dementia. They often occur years ahead of later symptoms. At this stage, it's common for the loved one living with dementia to forget things more often or have trouble remembering details about even familiar topics. Usually, the short-term memory such as recalling recent events and people met recently is impacted initially. Learning and retaining new information becomes more difficult. That's why asking repetitive questions is a hallmark of the disease as is writing reminder notes to themselves about things like where the car is parked. It's common to repeat comments and stories within minutes without realizing it. However, long-term memory, such as childhood memories usually remain normal.

Loved ones living with mild dementia have everyday life confusion. Additionally, they're easily distracted. They may find it hard to keep track of the time and miss appointments or favorite TV programs. Abstract thinking and making sound judgments become more difficult. They may lose the initiative to enjoy activities that were once pleasurable or routine. They may misplace objects regularly or store them in unusual places and forget where they put them.

Repetition and mistakes are obvious. An inability to form or store new memories causes a loss of immediate memory (what just happened). Forgetting appointments or routine tasks, losing things (or getting lost), and having trouble with names, directions or time becomes common.

Daily medications are sometimes taken and sometimes forgotten. A loved one may take a double dose of the same medication. Prescription medication refills are often overlooked.

Often a loved one in the mild dementia stage may seem to be acting unlike his or her old self. They may easily become irritable or angry when they feel embarrassed.

Mood swings are common and usually stem from frustration. Everyone has good days where the person you're concerned about seems unchanged and bad days when he or she is having trouble coping. This is most common in situations that are new, unusual or stressful. In the early mild stage, it's common to get lost, leave a stove burner on, lock one's self out of the car or house, or experience other such incidents.

What Worked for Us to Help Laura's Cognition

- When Laura's forgetfulness grew obvious, I accepted this as our new reality. I learned to expect more missed appointments, misplaced objects, forgotten names or errands, momentary confusion and the loss of conversational threads. In the larger scheme of life, these are minor irritants and not that important.

- I didn't make a big deal about mistakes or appearance quirks. I found that preserving pride and self-esteem was of paramount importance.
- I learned to respond to repeated questions or statements as if I was hearing them for the first time. Naturally, the wonderful tool of distraction by introducing a new subject would break the repetition cycle. Changing activities, location or rooms helped also.
- I learned to rely on lists, diaries, calendars and notebooks to compensate for Laura's memory glitches. We kept a large calendar in the kitchen and posted appointments and activities on it. It helped both of us.
- We discontinued supplements such as ginkgo biloba and vitamin E which a 2010 National Institutes of Health panel found to have no effect on memory. Although certain drugs approved for dementia may slow the rate of decline in some people, especially when started early, we chose to not utilize them because of possible gastrointestinal issues. Since Laura suffered life-long distress from periodic bouts of various intestinal issues, we were cautious of the foods, liquids and medications she consumed.
- Laura and I spend time together labeling names in old photos albums, organizing memorabilia, records, awards and doing other memory-based activities while we could. We continued enjoying several social bridge groups and periodic travel both to Europe and throughout the United States.
- Laura made mistakes with money, cooking, hobbies, housework and other activities. I downplayed the importance of her minor mistakes.
- Naturally, Laura's previously familiar activities sometimes caused her frustration, took longer or were done incorrectly. Her major trouble areas involved things that required multistep sequences, concentration, prioritizations, judgment and mathematical reasoning.

- For our entire married life, Laura balanced the checkbook and wrote checks to pay our bills but, now, I became involved in checkbook routine and double-checked expenditures and deposits. I watched especially for unrecorded or multiple payments for the same bill. Eventually, I took over all checkbook and bill paying duties.
- I removed Laura's credit cards from her purse and put them in my wallet.
- We both worked together to look for ways Laura could accomplish her favorite activities rather than give them up because it was now difficult to do them to her former standards.
- I encouraged the continued use of her longtime skills such as baking cookies, preparing meals and selecting clothes to wear every day. I helped her on these activities and she appreciated it.
- It was sometimes difficult but I resisted the urge to step in and do things for Laura. Rather, I tried to help her by allowing more time and minimizing any errors she made.
- Laura stopped reading books written by her favorite romance genre author. I downplayed this issue and stopped buying them as soon as they were released which was our former custom.

What Worked for Us to Help Laura's Emotional Health

- I found that fear and worry fed Laura's mood swings. Laura refused to talk about her onset of dementia but she was aware that something was not right. Sometimes Laura drew inward and other times she acted out with frustration and a shorter temper.
- I tried to not to mistake moodiness for rudeness. I accepted that a bad mood was a sign of Laura's struggle with dementia.

- I tried to encourage Laura to state her concerns: "Are you worried?" "Are you scared?" But I didn't force conversation if she cognitively retreated and became silent.

What Worked for Us to Help Laura's Physical Health

- Laura handled her own self-care, but I helped when minor issues arose.
- I gave Laura support which reinforced her abilities. Her functioning well extended self-reliance and independence.
- I relied more strongly on routine by shifting our daily activities so that dressing, grooming, meal times, getting out of the house, resting and bathing came about in the same order and time every day. I learned that habit and routine helped Laura's brain compensate.
- I organized our closets so everything had a place and kept it consistent. All the seldom used or out of season clothes were moved to spare closets. All the casual, flat shoes were stored in boxes together as were the dressy, flat shoes. Both were organized by color. Purses were organized similarly. The mid and high heeled shoes were kept together but moved to the spare closets as I discouraged her from wearing shoes with mid and high heels. Every storage container was marked with the contents. All of Laura's slacks were kept together as well as her shirts/blouses. All jackets were placed in one location. Everything was organized by casual and dressy. All expensive dresses were stored in the back of our master closet.
- Grab bars were placed for safety reasons at all entrance doors, adjacent to toilets, tub and shower entrances and lower level on the tub walls for sitting and standing assistance. We removed the glass door from the master shower and replaced it with a curtain. This facilitated the use of a shower extension wand and shower chair. This helped Laura

get used to them because they were needed later. Seniors have more falls in bathrooms than other places.

What Worked for Us to Help Laura's Social Life

- Denial of dementia has a common and strong social component. Laura's friends did not always see the subtle but increasing changes that I did. Or possibly they did not want to think of Laura's decline because it was difficult for them to accept also. No one likes declining health. Because the exact cause of dementia can't always be determined, some friends chose to act as though no impairment existed at all.
- I did my best to keep Laura socially engaged. We visited the homes of several close married friends each month, always calling them before we dropped in. They were a godsend as they seemed to realize what was occurring to Laura and understood her need to socialize.
- Family and friends did not know how to help unless I made specific requests. I found that what may look like obliviousness or refusal to help was often simple uncertainty. No one could read our minds. Most haven't dealt with dementia before but seemed to want to help in some way and did not feel being asked was an intrusion.
- Laura started to have lunch dates with her close lady friends regularly. The friend usually drove and I ensured expenses were shared by giving the friend Laura's credit card when she arrived. These one-on-one outings were amazingly helpful and the social stimulation worked its magic.
- I encouraged Laura's lifelong habit of keeping in telephone contact with distant family and friends. Saturday mornings were usually devoted to calling others and chatting.
- We visited our grandsons several afternoons each week, always taking some enjoyable fast food treat as their after-school snack. After a short visit, we would be off to a different adventure.

- Laura liked to shop. We visited both the higher end and bud-get ladies clothing stores fairly frequently. Laura liked to keep up with what was fashionable. Thankfully, she liked to look more than she did to buy.

Positive Affirmations

"Success is getting what you want. Happiness is wanting what you get." – *Dale Carnegie*

"Just one small positive thought in the morning can change your whole day." – *The Dalai Lama*

"We make a living by what we get, we make a life by what we give." – *Winston Churchill*

"It is under the greatest adversity that there exists the great-est potential for doing good, both for oneself and others." – *The Dalai Lama*

End Notes

[1]   https://www/caregiving.org/wp-content/uploads/2015/05/ 2015_caregivingintheUS_final-repoet-June4_web.pdf

[2]   https://www.caregiving.org/wp-content/uploads/2018/03/ coc-fact-sheet-12-taking-care-of-yourself.pdf

[3]   National Plan to Address Alzheimer's Disease, 2018 Update, 10/19/2018
https://aspe.hhs.gov/national-alzheimers-project-act

[4]   National Institute for Health (NIH) Research Summit on Alzheimer's Disease-Related Dementias was a two-day (March 14 and 15, 2019) meeting sponsored by the U. S. Department of Health and Human Services and private sector organizations.
https://videocast.nih.gov/resesearchsummit/March2019

[5]   Here is a list of the highest-level Alzheimer's Association International Conferences (AAIC) abstracts and press releases used to develop the ten-item summary:
AAIC 2019, Los Angeles, CA from July 14-18, 2019
AAIC 2018, Chicago, IL from July 21-25, 2018
AAIC 2017, London, England, from July 16-20, 2017
AAIC 2016, Toronto, Canada, from July 22-28, 2016
AAIC 2015, Washington, DC, from July 18-23, 2015
AAIC 2014, Copenhagen, Denmark, from July 12-17, 2014
AAIC 2013, Boston, MA, from July 13-18, 2013
AAIC 2012, Vancouver, British Columbia, from July 14-19, 2012
AAIC 2011, Paris, France, from July 16-21, 2011
AAIC 2010, Honolulu, Hawaii, from July 10-15, 2010
AAIC 2009, Vienna, Austria, from July 11-16, 2009
AAIC 2008, Chicago, Illinois, from July 26-31, 2008
AAIC 2007, Washington, DC, from June 9-12, 2007
AAIC 2006, Madrid, Spain, from July 15-20, 2006
AAIC 2004, Philadelphia, PA, from July 20-25, 2004
AAIC 2002, Stockholm, Sweden, July 20-25, 2002
AAIC 1998, Amsterdam, Netherlands, July 18-23, 1998

CHAPTER 21

Epilogue (Preview of Moderate Dementia)

"Compassion is the wish for another being to be free from suffering; love is wanting them to have happiness."
– The Dalai Lama

My book on the Tender Loving Care (TLC) Story relating to mild dementia ended with the last chapter. This epilogue is provided to furnish a preview of the moderate stage and summarize future TLC caregiving challenges.

The moderate stage is more challenging than the mild stage: Because the loved one living with dementia will experience more severe personal difficulties. These result in exhibiting behaviors that are much more challenging to the caregiver. My next book will address how Laura's behaviors became extremely challenging and how I overcame each difficulty using Tender Loving Care.

Laura was around 70 years old when she transitioned from mild to moderate dementia. Her physical health was excellent, probably the same as a 60-year-old senior woman. We kept traveling but modified our plans to include another close couple when we embarked on European travel adventures. They were both understanding and the wife helped Laura immensely with personal care tasks such as accessing toilet facilities in a foreign country. At this time, we had been married over 40 years. They were all good years and continued during Laura's moderate stage when I was astute enough to maintain my emphasis on Tender Loving Care.

Here is a summary of the chapters in *A Guide for Caregivers of Loved Ones in the Moderate Stage of Alzheimer's and Related Dementia Diseases*:

You will find my stories truly fascinating at times and extremely sad at other times. However, you will gain a complete understanding of how to use Tender Loving Care to help a loved one during their challenging moderate dementia years.

These cognitive challenges increase:

- Memory loss
- Disorientation
- Routine, practical and personal skills are lost
- Changing technology baffles your loved one
- Higher skills deteriorate
- Skills using the three R's are lost

These emotional challenges intensify:

- Personality changes
- Mood changes
- Sundowners
- Night-timers and night-terrors
- Sunrisers confusion
- Narcissism
- Confabulations
- Social withdrawal
- Apathy, impassivity and indifference
- Wanting to go home
- Dysphoria, depression, sadness, crying
- Euphoria, elation, laughing

- Pseudobulbar affect
- Agitation, irritability, anxiety, fear, stress
- Verbal aggression, shouting, screaming
- Physical aggression, slapping, punching, kicking, kneeing, biting, pinching, hair pulling

These physical challenges increase:

- Unsafe driving
- Walking, stair climbing, stair descending, balance
- Wandering inside
- Wandering outside
- Shadowing
- Repetitive behaviors, restlessness, rummaging

These complex and multiple (cognitive, emotional and physical) challenges begin:

- Delusions
- Hallucinations
- The mirror sign
- Misidentification syndrome
- Capgras syndrome

These simple, incremental Activities of Daily Living become overwhelmingly complex:

- Making the morning coffee
- Cooking
- Cleaning
- Operating common household appliances
- Using common tools
- Operating electronic devices

These basic Activities of Daily Living deteriorate:

- Transferring (getting out of a chair or a bed and standing upright)
- Walking
- Toileting
- Washing and bathing
- Personal hygiene and grooming
- Dressing
- Eating
- Drinking
- Resistance to care, uncooperativeness

The next book will continue the focus on using Tender Loving Care to overcome the challenging behaviors that are common in the moderate stage. I will explain what happened to Laura, give background information and tell what worked for us. You will be amazed and astounded by the loved one's moderate dementia experience. As in this mild dementia book, there will be a wealth of practical, common sense information provided. It was gleaned from my personal caregiving experience and over a decade of personal research into books, magazine articles and Internet sites devoted to Alzheimer's disease and related dementia diseases. It will be easy to understand and you will come away with a thorough knowledge of the moderate dementia phase. Becoming enlightened, empowered and filled with hope is the realistic objective of every caregiver providing Tender Loving Care to a loved one living with dementia.

This book is a love story. It is a story of the greatest possible love that can exist between two people. In this book, you will learn that Laura wants to kill Tom for his imagined horrendous behavior that only occurred in her hallucinations, Tom accepts Laura's perceived, untrue, mis-reality and returns her attempted murderous violence with love, care and compassion.

If attempted murder can be satisfactorily dealt with using Tender Loving Care, then certainly the other 50 or so challenging behaviors of the moderate stage can be resolved similarly. You will never regret reading the book titled *The TLC Story-Moderate Dementia | A Guide for Caregivers of Loved Ones in the Moderate Stage of Alzheimer's and Related Dementia Diseases.*

Made in USA - North Chelmsford, MA
1061550_9781734406405
03.23.2020 1006